# FIRST STEPS

# 2KETO

## Getting started with a ketogenic lifestyle

# IAN R PRATHER
# & JIM WITHERS

**First Steps 2 Keto**

First published in 2019 by

**Panoma Press Ltd**
48 St Vincent Drive, St Albans, Herts, AL1 5SJ, UK
info@panomapress.com
www.panomapress.com

Book layout by Neil Coe.

Printed on acid-free paper from managed forests.

**ISBN 978-1-784521-68-4**

# Dedication

This book is dedicated to every person who has been lost to poor health due to overconsumption of sugar.

# Acknowledgements

Special thanks to everyone at Panoma Press, especially Mindy Gibbins-Klein and Emma Herbert, for diligently working as mentors with us throughout the writing, editing, designing and marketing of this book. We would also like to thank them for finding value in our message and for helping us to make our vision a reality.

We would like to acknowledge Dr. Andy Lazris who provided information and permission to reprint information we found invaluable, as well as others who came before us to provide vital information, to utilize and help us form the substance of this book.

To the many enlightened doctors and medical professionals who have taken responsibility to get self-educated outside of an educational system that does not provide the same information that these amazing people are finding outside the system, we say thank you. You have shown us the need to be our own advocates as well. We appreciate all we have learned and continue to learn from you.

We would also like to thank all of the people who gave of their time to read and provide invaluable feedback on our book. We love and value them, and we appreciate the time they took to help make it better. To the online members of our Facebook groups, we also thank them for believing in our message and growing with us.

Jim would like to thank his wife, Tammy, and his family for all their support. Ian would like to also thank his wife, Betsy, for the innumerable times she has reviewed and edited this book, and for her dedication to ensuring it was finished at the last hour!

# Table of Contents

# CHAPTER 1

# Everyone Has Lost Someone to Poor Health

---

Fred R. Prather was an athlete in his youth back in the 1950s and 1960s. He married his high school sweetheart right after graduation from high school. Their first child, Ian, was born in December of 1968; followed by two sisters over the next three years.

Like many Americans of the time, Fred started smoking cigarettes as a young man. It was just the cool thing to do. For decades after and leading up to giant multibillion-dollar lawsuits against the tobacco companies, these companies insisted that cigarettes were safe, did not cause any harmful effects and were not addictive.

These companies absolutely knew of the health risks to people, and they also knew beyond a shadow of a doubt that nicotine is addictive. Once they had you hooked, they had a customer until they killed you. We have seen this same behavior repeated in other industries. One of those industries is the sugar industry.

Fred loved soda. Full sugar soda. In fact, he consumed 10 to 12 cans of soda per day. He drove around in a van for the A/C company he owned and it was a continuous running joke about all of the aluminum soda cans rolling around inside. Fred also loved Twinkies, Snowballs, Little Debbie's, and he loved drive-through windows.

Fred was the owner of Prather Air Conditioning Company. He was overweight, over-stressed and spent his days in hot attics. He was gone to work before the sun came up and still at work when the sun went down at night. Fred had a great sense of humor and comedic timing and kept everyone in stitches. His employees loved him and loved working for him. Fred was just an ordinary American man, building a business, providing for his family, and eating the way many did at that time. It would not be a stretch to say he was addicted to sugar and nicotine.

At the age of 32 years, Fred Robert Prather had his first heart attack. He was dropped off at the emergency room by his wife, Sue. I am sure he didn't even want to go. Sue dropped him at the door and went to park the car. As she rushed into the emergency room, instead of finding medical personnel frantically working to save his life, Sue found Fred standing at the counter filling out insurance forms. Sue grabbed Fred and shoved him through the doors of the emergency room screaming, "This man is having a heart attack!"

Having gotten everyone's attention, they went to work on Fred and were able to keep him alive, even after realizing he was filling out insurance forms with no pulse or detectable blood pressure. Fred survived what medical professionals at the time called a "young smoker's heart attack." He spent a fair amount of time in the hospital and even had to be evacuated from our town on the Texas Gulf Coast to Houston due to an approaching hurricane.

Fred and Sue were advised that he was just under too much stress from the pressures of running his own business. He was told if he didn't stop smoking cigarettes, lose some weight and stop taking in so much sugar that he would die. Sue took this extremely seriously and started cooking healthy meals for Fred. In came the salt substitute, the healthy heart cookbooks, and she did her part to help Fred change his habits.

Fred lived four more years.

Fred did take a partner in business to lower the stress levels. I have no idea if it did or not. What I do know, as his son aged 13 years, that a year before his death he took me deer hunting on an oil company lease up in central Texas. One of his best friends was an executive of that oil company and invited us up for a father/son hunt.

We barely made it out of the neighborhood when he pulled into the first convenience store that we saw. He told me to wait in the vehicle and when he returned he was tucking a pack of cigarettes into his pocket. He tossed a pouch of chewing tobacco (that mom had forbidden me to use) into my lap. Dad looked me right in the eyes, pointed his finger at me and said, "Don't you tell your mother I am smoking." I didn't.

Despite all the things I had heard my mother tell her friends and relatives when I was in earshot, I didn't tell her. Despite the fear I had of losing my larger than life dad, I didn't. I didn't say a word.

One year later, my dad left to go back to that same deer lease. I begged him to let me go. He simply said this time was for the grownups. He said, "Next time son, I promise." I remember crying as he left.

My dad never came home. His second heart attack was a widow maker. Fred Robert Prather died at 36 years of age in November of 1983, and I was 14 years old. There never was a "next time."

This still upsets me at the age of 50. What upsets me most is that I blamed myself for his death for many years after that. I punished myself for not telling my mom. I actually remember at dinner one night, during that last year of his life, my dad getting really angry and saying to my mother, "Sue, I have no idea why you are going to all this trouble to cook this healthy food because when I leave this house I stop at the first store I see and buy me some Twinkies and a Coke." I remember my mother saying something to the effect, "Well Fred, if you die, it won't be because I didn't do what I could to keep you alive."

Despite being told exactly what would happen if he didn't make the changes to his diet, reduce his weight and stop smoking cigarettes, Fred could not, would not, and did not stop or change. Exactly what the doctors told him would happen did happen. These addictive products were so powerful that even though doctors told him the truth, he could not, would not, and did not stop.

Fred Robert Prather died in Buffalo, Texas in November of 1983 just as his son started high school.

As difficult as it is to write this and to go through all of these painful memories again, please take a moment and think about the people you have lost in your life to personal decisions they have made about their health. Obesity, diabetes and heart disease have taken so many loved ones, friends, family members, coworkers and partners.

We couldn't write this book without including these memories of important people lost to us to these powerful health conditions caused by poor choices. It is unfortunate that big companies have obscured and manipulated the public, the government and the medical profession about the safety of their products.

Jim witnessed the death of two of his favorite uncles due to complications of diabetes. One of them passed after losing a leg to amputation, and the other after refusing amputation. The results were the same. Both of these important men that Jim loved died. Dietary choices to eat foods full of sugar caused each of these men to lose control of their blood sugar.

Their blood sugar got worse and worse until even the medications, including insulin, failed to work. Jim witnessed with his own eyes two of his favorite uncles die horrible deaths. Here is more on Jim's experience:

My grandfather migrated from Oklahoma to Northern California during the 1930s, seeking work like most of the nation during that time. His family picked fruit in orchards and literally camped and slept on the side of the road. This is the life his four sons grew up in and all of them wanted to escape. Uncle Alan volunteered for the U.S. Army and was deployed to Vietnam. When he returned, Uncle Alan never spoke a word about his experience there. It became obvious to everyone that he would never be the same.

Uncle Alan was the first adult to ever treat Jim as an equal, even when Jim was still a kid. Uncle Alan always had a mischievous gleam in his eye and an infectious grin. He also always had a beer in his hand. Back in those days, it seemed to be one of the few ways to cope with the horrors of war. We continue to see this even today. We call it PTSD.

Drinking and driving resulted in Uncle Alan spending over 10 years in jail. When he finally got some help in his late 50s and early 60s for his demons from war, the physical devastation caused by the Standard American Diet and all the carbs from the continuous beer he consumed every waking hour had taken a toll on his body and he was so unhealthy that he was confined to a wheelchair.

In 2017, Uncle Alan fell out of that wheelchair and received a deep wound to his right leg. He was a stubborn man and refused medical treatment until he became delirious with fever from the infection that ultimately got into his bloodstream. After being admitted to the hospital, Uncle Alan refused to allow them to amputate his leg.

Jim visited his favorite Uncle Alan for three consecutive days hoping and praying he would wake up. Jim wanted to let him know how much he loved him. Uncle Alan never regained consciousness. He passed away in that hospital bed due to the complications of type 2 diabetes. He died of a dietary disease of personal choice that could have been prevented.

Hearing these stories, a person could hope that we would have learned the lessons these men failed to learn and would have seen the error of their ways, going on to make much better personal choices about our health. This is **not** what happened. We ended up following these men down the same exact path to obesity and diabetes. We ate the same food and got the same results.

Jim lived through his first heart attack. Ian added a consistent three pounds per year from the age of 21 to the age of 45 when he weighed 250 pounds. A new company doctor who threatened Ian with his employment shocked him into seeking better information and making some changes.

Perhaps it is the grace of being righteous men, as Jim so eloquently describes, "The only difference between an unrighteous man and a righteous man is that the righteous man gets up one more time when he falls." Ian and Jim both decided to rise up. Somehow and for some reason, we got up one more time. In a moment of desperation and fear, we opened up to some better information. Why? Neither one of us has a good answer for that.

Jim lost most of his right foot due to amputation from the results of the symptoms of diabetes. Many people could and have gotten bitter and angry at the world. Jim will tell you today that losing most of his foot is the best thing that ever happened to him.

Perhaps better information was available when we became open to seeking it. We really don't know but we agree that knowing what we now know, we believe 100% that the deaths of those close to us were deaths that were preventable. We have also researched and learned enough to firmly believe the only reason that people aren't in jail and these companies responsible for this shut down and put out of business is because they kill people slowly enough. If it happened a little faster, perhaps it would be criminal.

The fact is we lost some people we love and almost lost ourselves over illness caused by dietary choices. Illness that most doctors are just managing with medication. The absolute failure to address the root cause of this dietary disease is what is killing people slowly. We call this the *sugar agenda*.

The government continues to get the big money from big businesses, the big businesses continue to control the medical schools and what they teach. The doctors who come into the modern system have the kickbacks and payoffs from big pharma built into the compensation system for simply continuing to prescribe the drugs that manage the symptoms that are *caused* by the foods we have been told to eat by the government. The giant wheel keeps turning while the public gets ground to dust by the system. Two ordinary guys hope to change this, one person at a time.

## Type 2 diabetes and insulin

There are two types of diabetes – type 1 and type 2 – and we do not want in any way to discount the fact that some human beings have a pancreas that simply does not produce insulin, or enough insulin. This type 1 diabetic must inject insulin to control blood sugar. These type 1 diabetics will be insulin dependent, through no fault of their own, for life unless there is advancement in the field of pancreas regeneration or some amazing advances in technology.

We believe the majority of type 2 diabetes is a result of **dietary choice**. The result is an increasing lack of blood sugar control (the sugar roller coaster) that is caused by the ever-increasing consumption of sugar/carbs to the point at which the system ceases to function properly. Unless there is some other condition causing the pancreas to fail in producing enough insulin to control blood sugar, type 2 diabetes is a dietary choice.

This book is not an argument that other possibilities don't exist. Instead we will focus on the vast majority of people that we have personally worked with and introduced to the ketogenic lifestyle and the results we have seen.

We believe that the addition of insulin into this situation is the exact example of treating a dietary-choice illness with medication instead of dealing with the root cause of the problem, which is the overconsumption of sugar. We believe, due to what we have personally experienced, that type 2 diabetics who start injecting insulin, instead of stopping the ever-increasing consumption of sugar, is simply making the problem worse. This is like fighting a forest fire with a flame thrower instead of just putting the fire out.

Unfortunately, this is recommended treatment from the medical field. First drugs like Metformin, then Glipizide, and then ultimately insulin injections are prescribed to control blood sugar.

Unless a person has some issue of a continuing deterioration of pancreas function that is separate and apart from the overconsumption of sugar, we simply point out that this **dietary choice** to continue to overconsume sugar is what causes blood sugar to go out of control. That is the root cause of this dietary illness.

Why doesn't the government, or the big associations involved with issues of diabetes, point out the glaring fact that people suffering the symptoms of type 2 diabetes should stop the wrong dietary choice of putting more sugar in the body? We suggest these type 2 diabetics should deal with the root cause of the problem instead of just medicating the symptoms.

If a person's blood sugar is out of control, **stop putting sugar in the system**.

## The business of insulin

In the year 2017, the insulin market was $42 billion. It is projected to increase by 8.8% by 2023. North America accounts for a 39.2% share of this number. This is a simple illustration that what we are eating on the Standard American Diet is damaging Americans worse than the rest of the world.

Americans are leading the world in numbers of people diagnosed with type 2 diabetes. Americans consume the most sugar and diagnose the most diabetes. There are other countries that have adopted our foods. They are rapidly catching up with us.

We simply have to ask, "How is that Standard American Diet working for you?" The truth is that the Standard American Diet has never worked for Americans and it is proving to have the same results on any person, group, or country that eats this way over the long term.

The number of global diabetic patients is rising at an astronomical pace. It has risen from **108** million in 1980 to **422** million in 2014 and it is expected to rise to **592** million by 2035. Globally, the International Diabetes Federation states that **425** million humans had diabetes in 2017 and this number is expected to reach **629** million by 2045.

Of course, the large pharmaceutical companies are rising to the occasion by gaining approval for more and more insulin pen type devices that make administering insulin injections super simple and virtually painless, making the entire process more simplified. Isn't that convenient?

No one seems interested in addressing the overconsumption of sugar and carbs. That is what is causing all this, especially in countries outside the USA that are moving as fast as they can to consume as much sugar as we do here, and they are getting the exact same results in obesity, heart disease and type 2 diabetes. There just isn't any profit to be made in actually addressing the root cause of this global crisis.

Here is a mind-boggling statistic:

Only **5%** of all diabetics are **type 1**. This means that **95%** of diabetics are *choosing* to have **type 2** diabetes based on the food they are eating. The government, big food, big pharma and most of the medical establishment seem perfectly content to keep prescribing Metformin, Glipizide and ultimately insulin to control blood sugar.

Why are they not telling this massive group of people to stop putting sugar in their body? The answer is **money**. It seems that nobody is willing to stand up to this system.

We have been honest enough with ourselves to ask the question: How in this world can two regular guys stand up to a decades-old system involving government, big pharma, big food, the education system, as well as the medical community? Add to that the media putting out and repeating some of the most ridiculous news stories about the ketogenic lifestyle.

The average person stays confused and manipulated by the system. They just don't know who to believe. Health and dietary issues have seemed to become another topic like politics. Keep repeating a lie often enough until it becomes the "truth." The public suffers. Our only hope is to keep sharing our truth and change one person at a time.

It is not an easy task to write a book like this, concerning these topics, and not sound like two guys on a rant about conspiracy theories. We want to share with you the truth we have experienced personally with our own health, as well as the truth we have now seen repeated in many other people who follow us. When they made the choice to minimize the intake of sugar, they changed their life and health, just as we did. They chose the ketogenic lifestyle. Ketogenic lifestyle? What does that even mean?

The ketogenic lifestyle is a way of eating that minimizes sugar (carbs), promotes a moderate intake of protein and a higher content of healthy fat. Just like our ancestors ate, up until a couple hundred years ago, when the sugar industry started mass production. This mass production drove the price down and enabled the sugar industry to start providing cheaper sugar to more people. Over this short period of time in human history, the average consumption of sugar has increased to the level that the human body is unable to process. The system begins to lose control and the medical community starts prescribing medications to control it instead.

There is written history dating back 2,500 years with fasting being used as a treatment for seizures. The ketogenic way of eating mimics the results of fasting in the production of ketones. The human body is designed to operate using ketones for fuel at the cellular level. The human body is also able to utilize glucose, or sugar, for energy. We are designed to operate in this hybrid way.

When body fat is released into the bloodstream, it undergoes processing in the liver that converts these fatty acids into three different types of ketone bodies: BHB (Beta-hydroxybutyric acid), Acetoacetate (AcAc) and Acetone. These ketones circulate in the bloodstream and enter the cells of the body to create energy, just as glucose does, even crossing the blood/brain barrier.

Some of the benefits reported of the ketogenic way of eating are:

*Weight loss

*Appetite control

*Mental focus/clarity/cognition benefits due to neuro-protective properties of ketones

*Increased energy

*Effective in *reversing* the symptoms of type 2 diabetes by minimizing sugar intake

*Lower blood pressure

*Powerful anti-inflammatory properties

We want to caution that anyone with medical issues or on prescription medication for blood pressure, blood sugar, or any other medical issue *must* work with their personal doctor and monitor these issues more closely than normal as we have seen the minimization of sugar cause big changes in ourselves and those we work with.

The ketogenic way of eating has become a very popular topic for several years now. While there have been some low-carb fads since the 1970s, there has never been such a sustained period of time in which interest in the ketogenic lifestyle has been this high or long. We feel that we are on the verge of a tipping point in understanding not only what ketogenic eating really is, but of mainstream America and the rest of the world waking up to the history of the sugar agenda, or the vast majority of humans will accept being fitted with an insulin pump so we can keep eating the way we do.

While there are many issues of concern for the media and political figures such as global warming and others, we strongly believe that changing the course now of the obscene amount of sugar ingested by the average human being would be the single most effective issue that would affect the health and wellness of millions of people **immediately.**

The staggering amount of money we are spending yearly for equipment and drugs to control blood sugar, or to pay the costs of the resulting obesity, heart and other medical problems that go hand in hand with consuming too much sugar, could actually be put to much better use to improve the world we live in.

# CHAPTER 2

# Take Responsibility for Your Own Health: It's Not Too Late to Live Your Best Life!

---

We made the decision to work together and share personal experience in writing this book. Although Jim is in California and Ian in Texas, we utilized technology to work together to produce the book you are now reading. For simplicity's sake, and with the reader in mind, we will use the word "we" to describe this collaboration in the rest of the book and we use individual names as needed.

We want to do our very best to allow you to get to know who we are as people. It is our true desire to share some simple steps we have learned and put into practice that may very well change your life and health for the better. The only way to know if the ketogenic lifestyle is for you is to do an honest test.

We want you to understand that we are not highly educated nutritionists. We are not doctors. We do not prescribe medications or claim to cure anything. We have both been talked down to and treated like we were stupid as we started our own personal ketogenic journey, and we have made the decision to never treat other people that way. We decided to create something that we wished had existed when we started.

We are just two regular guys who ate the Standard American Diet, just as the government, big food companies and big pharma have taught us to do, for all of our lives. It nearly killed us both. It doesn't kill people all at once but slowly over the years. We got fatter, less healthy and then achieved the amazing gift of type 2 diabetes. Here is some of our story to get to know us and the experience we have lived.

# Jim Withers

It was not until Jim lost most of his right foot as a symptom of diabetes that something changed in his thinking and mindset. Jim had been diabetic for 10 years, dependent on insulin, Glipizide and Metformin, but could not get his blood sugar under 300. Jim's doctors told him he would have to take these medications for the rest of his life because type 2 diabetes is a progressive lifelong disease.

Approximately two years ago, Jim stepped on a stone while chasing his little dog into the road when she escaped out the front door. This injury to the bottom of his right foot got infected and would not heal due to complications of his diabetes. Jim ended up in the hospital three days later. The infection had moved from the bottom of his foot all the way through to the top, and the doctors made the decision to remove infected areas of the foot to attempt to save it.

Because of this procedure, Jim was confined to his chair for six months. The doctors then came to realize that the infection had moved into the bones of his foot. Two toes were amputated first to attempt to remove the infection. This surgery confined Jim to his chair for an additional six months.

These surgeries caused a change in the wear pattern on the bottom of Jim's foot resulting in diabetic ulcers and ultimately the amputation of the front of Jim's right foot, and an additional six months confined to a chair.

Eighteen months confined to a chair is a lot of time to think about things and gave Jim ample time to take an inventory of his life. Jim took a hard look at what got him there, about his two uncles he had lost to diabetes, and about his own father who had been on insulin for almost 20 years. Was diabetes hereditary?

As a young man, he had no problem eating whatever he wanted. Jim always stayed right around 160 pounds. In the Navy he ate the chow the Navy fed him, trusting in the food pyramid way of eating because the Navy followed the ratios of protein, a vegetable, a starch, a fruit, and of course dessert.

In his mid- to late-20s, he gained an extra 40 pounds but he still looked okay as everyone was saying he needed to add a little meat on his bones. During the next 10 years in the Navy, Jim continued to gain weight until he was 20 pounds overweight. Jim was in his 30s.

Jim was instructed to exercise more and begin the standard low-fat diet, watching his portions, and keeping to his diet with no snacks. He did what they told him to do.

Sometime during this process, Jim came across some different information that said he should eat several small meals six or seven times a day. This is supposed to burn up more calories and speed up the metabolism. Jim went on to test the latest conventional wisdom and fad diets for years of yo-yo dieting.

By his mid-30s, Jim was 60 pounds overweight, and when he left the Navy he was diagnosed with type 2 diabetes. The VA prescribed a Metformin pill to help control his blood sugar. As time went on, Jim gained a little more weight and had to increase his medication to keep his diabetes under control. The next step was to go see the VA nutritionist who put Jim on the American Diabetes Association Diet. Jim continued to gain weight and require more medication. The doctors at the VA started adding different medications like Glipizide in addition to Metformin.

By his late 40s, the VA doctors prescribed insulin. Jim was taught to monitor his blood sugar with a glucose meter. He was still eating an ADA recommended diet and was instructed to see an endocrinologist who prescribed a short-acting insulin. Next came the long-acting insulin to better control his blood sugar. The "progressive" and "lifelong" disease was proving itself to be exactly that.

Even using all this prescribed medication, Jim's blood sugar was completely out of control. From a high in the 300s, it would drop down into the 30s or 40s and Jim would have to take in sugar to raise it back up. His blood sugar was like a roller coaster ride. Jim's health deteriorated to the point of feeling bad all the time. He had thrown in the towel on trying to diet perfectly. It seemed that nothing he did was helping. He started giving in to the overwhelming urges and cravings for sugar and starches. By age 52, Jim's feet started getting infected with diabetic ulcers and he was constantly ill.

Shortly after Jim was prescribed blood pressure medication, he had a heart attack. He was wondering if he was lucky to be alive at this point. It wasn't long after the heart attack that Jim chased his little dog out into the street.

After being confined to his chair for 18 months, thinking about all of this history, Jim started to realize that the "advice" he had been receiving about his health was incorrect. Although he had followed all of the recommendations given to him from the doctors, Jim came to the realization that what he was doing simply was not working. At a deep-down gut level Jim knew that if something didn't change, his life was over.

Jim became open to different and better information and was introduced to the ketogenic lifestyle by a friend named Dr. Robert Shapiro. This introduction was a game-changer in Jim's life and opened his eyes to a whole new way of eating that he did not know existed. Jim started to do his own research and became his own advocate and began to learn what worked for him. He actually started to get excited about life for the first time in many years.

Who could say what would have happened had he not been introduced to the ketogenic lifestyle? Jim finally came to the realization that he "didn't know what he didn't know."

For the first time in all the years of doctor's orders, prescriptions, and increasing numbers of medications, he actually made the one change that nobody in his previous experience had suggested: **Jim stopped eating sugar**.

It seems so simple today looking back, and it's incredible that it took what it did to get Jim to the place of understanding this simple idea. **Sugar is the devil.** It is a simple statement for Jim and 100% true. Jim had to start treating sugar like poison.

Jim asked himself the question he had never before considered. If his system could not control his blood sugar, and the ever-increasing amount of medications he was prescribed could not control his blood sugar, why in the world did Jim keep putting the one thing into his body that nothing could control? For a couple of years now, Jim has minimized the amount of sugar/carbs that go into his body and here is what has changed:

Jim is **medication free** now. Yes, you read that correctly. He does not take the 30 plus prescription medications, including

Metformin, Glipizide and two different types of insulin, that he previously took to control his blood sugar. Jim's blood pressure and weight are now normal and healthy. Jim now eats as his hunter gatherer ancestors did. We were designed to eat ketogenic, and having put ketogenic eating into practice, Jim is now healthier thanhe has been in decades. Once the sugar/carbs were removed, his body showed an amazing ability to heal.

By minimizing sugar/carb intake, Jim found his blood sugar dropping and his hunger and cravings were not so strong. This was the first time his blood sugar had dropped that was not due to using insulin.

We recommend to anyone on any type of medication to work closely with their personal doctor on issues of medication. It stands to reason that when we reduce the sugar going into the body, the amount of medications needed to control blood sugar will also be reduced. Each person is different and eating ketogenic can change things.

Jim started feeling better. After feeling as bad as he had felt for as long as he had, the realization that he was feeling so much better was almost like a spiritual awakening. Jim's mind certainly woke up, and he started researching and reading anything he could find about the ketogenic lifestyle.

He began taking simple steps like removing the tempting foods out of the house, cutting back and minimizing the amount of carbs/ sugar he put into his body, and paying attention to the amounts of fat and protein he was eating. Jim was simply amazed at how fast his health was returning. What he did not expect was some of the negative feedback he received.

Even as Jim was healing and changing right in front of their eyes, Jim had to endure other people's opinions about his lifestyle choices. It is a difficult thing to attempt to overcome a lifetime of incorrect programming as provided by the government, the food industry, the medical industry and the drug industry. Add to that having to deal with the incorrect programming of family members and friends, it is an amazing accomplishment for any of us to make the needed lifestyle change.

Jim heard comments about "eating all that fat," and that he was going to "die of a heart attack" if he kept eating that way. People in his life told him he was crazy. Jim knew on a deep-down, gut level that the choices he was making were the right thing for him. He knew he had to take responsibility for improving his own health, but he was questioned by friends and family about the long-term effects of this crazy "diet" he was doing. "Aren't you on cholesterol medication and blood pressure pills? Are you trying to kill yourself?"

These are the kinds of questions Jim faced, even while healing, yet it is interesting to note that for all those years, decades in fact, as Jim had become more obese, more unhealthy, more diabetic, and taking more and more medications, *nobody* said a word except the doctors who gave the standard advice, "Jim, you need to exercise more, and here is another prescription."

Jim stuck to his new lifestyle like his life depended on it. The first result was no longer needing his slow-acting insulin to control his blood sugar. It is mind-boggling now to look back and try to understand what was so difficult to accept about this concept.

When Jim stopped putting sugar in his body, his blood sugar actually controlled itself, yet not a single doctor had ever suggested this approach. After about three more weeks, Jim had to stop using his fast-acting insulin. If he did use it, his blood sugar plummeted extremely low because there was no longer an excessive amount of sugar in his blood to control.

Once again, we recommend working closely with your personal doctor on any issues of medications of this nature and this is a clear example of why.

As Jim stayed the course with the ketogenic lifestyle, he found he no longer needed Metformin or Glipizide for blood sugar control. As he stopped putting the sugar in his body, his body started healing and working properly again. With his blood pressure steadily coming down, Jim had to stop taking blood pressure medicine to keep it from going too low. This was another medication that was no longer needed simply by minimizing the amount of sugar/carbs he was ingesting.

What Jim had begun demonstrating to himself and others around him was that the ketogenic way of eating, just as our ancestors have done, was the single best choice he had made for his health.

What Jim could not understand was why nobody had ever suggested the approach of removing sugar/carbs in the first place. It seemed like such a simple concept that never occurred to him until his introduction to Dr. Shapiro.

Jim simply ignored any negativity from other people and decided to let results be his determining factor on issues of his personal health. With health returning, Jim became his own health advocate and started digging into the history of what has brought the entire world to this epidemic of diabetes, obesity and heart disease, and why he wasn't told to stop eating sugar.

## Ian Prather

Ian was headed down a very similar path as Jim was. Having worked for 25 years in the chemical industry, working rotating 12-hour shifts, Ian had steadily gained around three pounds per year. It doesn't sound like much, but that was from a starting weight of 185 pounds at the age of 21. By the age of 43, at five feet eight inches tall, Ian weighed in at 250 pounds. His t-shirt size was XXXL.

Ian had an old country company doctor who just overlooked things. He may have joked once or twice during annual physicals that it was time to say "no" to Blue Bell ice cream once in a while. It was always said jokingly and wasn't taken seriously. Ian knew of coworkers with high blood pressure or poor lung capacity, but these issues were jokingly brushed over. These issues could always wait until the annual physical next year.

That old country doctor finally retired, and the new company doctor was a retired Lt. Colonel from the United States Air Force. He was a very fit triathlete and the same age as Ian, 43 years old. Rumors started going around the plant that this new doctor was sending people home if they couldn't pass the annual physical to his personal requirements. He would demand a visit to the employee's personal physician and a written action plan to address obesity, blood pressure, lung capacity, or any other issue not up to his standard.

At Ian's annual physical he was informed for the first time ever that he was considered morbidly obese, in addition to terrible cholesterol and super high triglyceride numbers, horrible liver enzymes indicating inflammation, and ultimately a diagnosis of fatty liver and fasted blood sugar that would not come down below 120. Ian had the type of excess body fat, lipid profile, blood sugar and inflammation that causes humans to drop dead from heart attack or stroke. Just as his father had at age 36.

This same story repeated with about 33% of employees being confronted with some type of health issue that made them unfit for work in the opinion of the new company doctor. What we had wondered were just rumors became fact as employees we personally knew were sent home. Ian, who had always been confident in his abilities and was a highly rated back-up team leader, for the first time in 25 years felt his employment was under threat due to his physical health.

Ian worked huge amounts of overtime, basically living at the plant and sleeping at home. He wondered when he was supposed to "get more exercise?"

It's never an easy thing to be confronted with the truth about our weight or health, especially when we know deep down that we have failed ourselves, knowing that we have failed to take the personal responsibility necessary on a daily basis to keep ourselves healthy.

Ian had given in to the story we tell ourselves that we are just too busy. We give in to the convenience all around us that makes acquiring great tasting but unhealthy foods so fast and easy. We abdicate the personal responsibility for what we eat and slowly pay the price over time. Believe it or not, it is *exactly* the way the fast food corporations have designed things to work. Their goal is not to keep you healthy. Their goal is to design foods that make you crave more. Their goal is to make profit.

The truth is, like a majority of other Americans and other humans from countries around the world, we all have the excuses of being busy, working too much, or not having enough time. It's so much easier to choose convenience and speed. It is especially easy when what they are serving at drive-through windows all across the land tastes so *good!!* Exactly the way the marketing plans are designed. When we actually research the science that these billion-dollar companies use to create these marketing plans, the average person just doesn't have a chance.

Ian and Jim both had wake-up calls. Health crisis and fear of losing employment can be a motivating factor. Unfortunately, it takes this kind of a shock for most people to have a shift in the mindset and thinking required to make changes to improve personal health and wellness. It is our goal to help you bypass this drama and get better information to make a personal change faster than we did.

For some, even the life events mentioned above are not enough to overcome the habits we have built over our lifetimes. Sadly, many are so addicted to sugar and the release of the pleasure chemicals caused by eating "comfort food," they end up paying the ultimate price of even more serious health issues, including heart attack, stroke, and even death.

We both had serious wake-up calls. We had an awakening that caused us to start questioning everything. We started researching, learning, and became open minded to the fact that many others had taken the same path of the Standard American Diet and food pyramid and arrived at the same unhealthy results.

We also came to understand that the system is not addressing the root cause of the problem. That root cause is the overconsumption of sugar/carbs in the western diet, overconsumption to the point that we are totally overwhelming our body's system that controls our blood sugar. After being overwhelmed and overworked, the system just stops functioning properly.

Ian did what many would do in the same circumstances feeling their livelihood was threatened. He got a gym membership. He committed to going an hour before or after work six days a week. After floundering around in the gym for six months, Ian's weight was exactly the same. The next annual physical was six months away.

Ian decided to hire a coach, and this decision to work with a trainer was not an easy one. It was expensive. During the interview process, the coach inquired if Ian cooked at all. Nope, not ever.

"That changes today. You will eat what I tell you to eat, when I tell you to eat it, and you will prepare and cook meals every day. If you are not willing to do this, we have nothing else to discuss," said the coach.

Out of desperation, Ian agreed, and over the course of the next few years, this single decision to finally take responsibility for personal health changed *everything* in his life.

Each of us has to get to that place for ourselves. We have to open our minds up to better information than what we have blindly accepted in the past. Our goal and our hope is that we can shorten that process to understanding. The very best time to take responsibility for your own health and wellness is today. You do not have to get so far down the road of obesity, heart disease and diabetes as we did.

It has been said that "insanity is doing the same thing over and over and expecting different results" and it became clear that to get different results, Ian and Jim were going to have to make some changes. If you want to stop getting the same results, you have to stop doing what produced those results. They both decided it was time to become their own advocates because doing what they learned before had not produced the results of better health and wellness.

We have had to battle some myths about ketogenic eating. Years later, the same myths continue to be told by people or industries who have a financial interest in keeping us sick as long as possible because it's more *profitable*. From the celebrity trainer talking negatively about ketogenic eating because it gets them attention in the media, to the doctor or scientist putting out information, or studies funded by the big food industry or big pharma that magically produce the results favorable to those paying for the studies, we continue to witness these tactics over and over again. Once again, as in politics, when a lie is repeated often enough it becomes the accepted truth.

We continue to hear the myths such as the idea a person has to give up all the foods they love. We hear that we can't eat bread or pasta or desserts. No more eating pizza or pancakes, and eating ketogenic is impossible while one is on the road or traveling. "It's just too hard. It's not sustainable long term. All that fat just isn't healthy." We have heard it all. The real whopper is hearing medical professionals say you need sugar!

There is no such thing as an essential carbohydrate. Our bodies are 100% capable of creating the small amount of glucose it may need. However, the truth is that big food companies are putting sugar in *everything* and the government is allowing them to camouflage the fact by allowing them to use *56 different names for sugar.*

We have seen some nutrition labels that actually use *four* different names for sugar, yet never use the word sugar on the package. Unless the average person happens to know all 56 different names for sugar, how would they possibly know what they are eating?

It is this quantity of sugar that the average human is now ingesting that is the root cause of the major escalation of the health crisis we are now seeing with obesity, heart disease and diabetes. In our research, we have learned that in the late 1700s the average person consumed **one** 12 oz. can of soda worth of sugar **every seven days.** Today, the average person consumes this much sugar **every seven hours**.

We cannot stress enough how important it is for you to understand that the human body, as amazing and adaptable as it can seem, is simply not designed to process this amount of sugar. Anyone who tells you otherwise is either completely oblivious, does not care about you as a human being, or is only interested in making money.

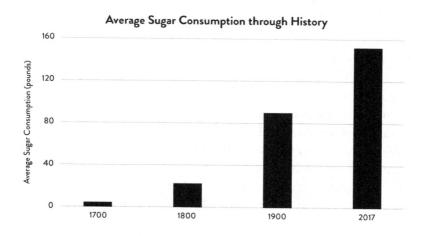

Average Sugar Consumption through History

It does not take a giant leap of understanding for a couple of regular guys to see these previous numbers of a drastic increase of sugar consumption over the past 200 years and the following image concerning the increase in people diagnosed with diabetes in just the last 30 years to understand one simple fact: the more sugar is consumed, the higher the diagnosis of diabetes.

The higher the incidence of diabetes, you will also find similar trends in obesity and heart disease. This is the trifecta of damage caused by overconsumption of sugar.

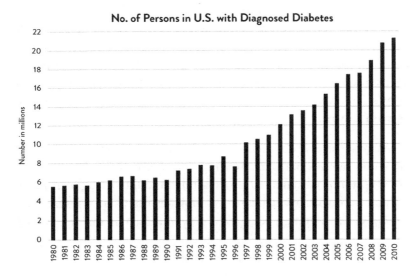

No. of Persons in U.S. with Diagnosed Diabetes

We have also seen not only in our own personal health but in many others we have worked with, that when we minimize and eliminate sugar, these numbers turn around. We see people reducing and eliminating medications needed to control blood sugar, blood pressure, cholesterol, and other medications of this type. We also believe that this is the beginning. We are just getting started and want to create such a groundswell of positive results and benefits that we can no longer be ignored and no longer accept the status quo. A huge part of the ketogenic lifestyle is getting better educated.

We are learning that this is simply an educational process of learning what foods and ingredients cause an elevation in blood glucose (sugar) and what foods and ingredients we can exchange out to stop the elevation of blood sugar.

In these modern times, we have found these foods and ingredients to be so much more readily available that acquiring them is nothing more than an excuse. We also believe that anyone that uses *expense* as an excuse needs to seriously reevaluate their priorities. We make no apologies for it, just as we no longer make excuses.

Obesity, heart disease, diabetes, and all the treatments and medications for these issues are what is expensive. What is the cost of not being there for your partner, your children, or your grandkids? Taking the responsibility to eat foods that avoid all these health issues is an investment in actual healthcare as opposed to continuing to pay the consequences of poor dietary choices. We call the costs of these poor choices "paying for sick care." Our goal is to reverse this mindset with some basic education.

We have learned that making excuses about being too busy to cook, while very true for some, can also just be a cop-out. Even if you are one of those super busy people, or someone who travels a great deal, the good news is that with a little planning you will have no issue eating ketogenic on the road. It is also a matter of priorities to do some meal prep in advance to save time during the week. It is simply a matter of creating new habits and taking responsibility for what we eat.

You will hear it from us, over and over again, the subject of personal responsibility. We are all witnesses of what leaving this responsibility to the government, big food companies, fast food companies, and big pharma have done for our health. We must choose to get better educated and make our personal health and wellness a priority.

Getting rid of old destructive habits and acquiring new and healthier habits is simply a choice we make to practice new ideas. Building these new habits is just practice. Just as we get better at anything in life that we do, it is practice that causes the improvement. The simple fact remains that we had to get started somewhere, and our goal is to help you get started too.

One of the first changes in mindset we had to develop is that *ketogenic eating is a lifestyle choice, not a diet.*

We have experienced too many times the person who eats ketogenic and gets great results while doing so. For whatever reason they go back to their non-ketogenic way of eating and get the exact same results they always have. Obesity, heart disease, high blood pressure and diabetes.

We then hear how the ketogenic lifestyle just didn't work for them. This demonstrates how powerful and evil sugar is to humans. The ketogenic lifestyle absolutely works when we practice it, just as continuing to eat the way we always have works exactly the opposite.

Although some people "go keto" to drop a few pounds for vacation or some event, when they "go off keto" the weight comes right back on and then some. Why is that? Consuming carbs can cause us to retain water. For all the fast results we see bragged about with some people describing losing 10 pounds in a week by "going keto," the truth is that most of this would be water weight.

As fast as water weight comes off when sugar/carbs are removed from what we eat, that water weight comes right back on when the sugar/carbs are added back. This is simply a scientific reality. For every gram of sugar/carb we eat, the body can retain up to four grams of water.

Another issue that we will touch on now but take a deeper dive into later is really very simple: the human body is not designed to process the quantity of sugar that the average human is now consuming on a daily basis. Our systems are overloaded. Food companies are putting sugar into everything and most average humans have no idea how much sugar they ingest on a daily basis.

Most average people have no idea how that sugar affects the body, or that the hormone insulin has the job to get that spike in blood sugar back down to "normal." Most have no idea that for the vast majority of people their blood sugar is out of control. The system is broken. More on this later.

We are all too busy! Too busy eating what tastes good, and too busy to cook or pay attention to ingredients. Too busy to read labels. It can seem like such a hassle. It's so much easier to just hit the drive-through window and get everyone exactly what they want in minutes! And the food tastes so good!! This is exactly the way the big fast food companies have designed their foods.

It could be an entirely separate book to go into the detail of the science behind fast food, how it is designed to make us crave it, and how the marketing behind it starts with children. Once you become your own advocate and start paying attention to their methods, it is shocking and frightening seeing the control this marketing has over human beings. Especially moms.

Many of the wives/partners, moms and grandmothers are too busy trying to keep everyone they take care of happy and fed. Women wear so many different hats each day and we salute them for being amazing. But when it comes to feeding the family, it is so easy to allow convenience to win out due to the busy and hectic schedule that many people face. It is so much simpler to just feed them what they want. The convenience of drive-through windows in just about any town makes it possible for everyone to have exactly what they want in minutes.

This does not mean that the food choices anyone is making are in any way healthy, and this single habit, made for the sake of efficiency, is one of the most horrible things we are doing to ourselves and our families. We understand that you are busy. We also understand that when you get better educated on the costs of making decisions like this based on efficiency, from being in a hurry and due to the convenience provided, we believe the moms and grandmothers of this world will decide it's simply not worth it.

We believe it is going to be this very group of women who ultimately lead themselves, their partners, their children and grandchildren into a direction of better health and wellness. We are absolutely convinced this is starting to happen now. This is truly a hope and goal that this book effectively speeds up the process.

We believe that this group of moms and grandmothers will be at the forefront of change in the health and wellness of the world. You will be an example to your partner, your children and your grandchildren. It will be moms and grandmothers that change the health of the world.

No offense meant to the men who cook for the family or partners. You have a choice as well to take responsibility for yourself and lead those you cook for to better health and wellness. We have come to realize you are important, but the reality is that the group of wives/partners, moms and grandmothers make up the vast majority of the audience we have been personally working with and we acknowledge this fact.

We want to make a point with this book that we literally have the power to choose a healthy weight. We have the power to choose to feel better. We have the power to choose to put into practice better habits. We have the power to stop making excuses that keep us sick and make us sicker. We have the power to examine our personal history, and the history of government actions as well as the history of businesses and individuals who have shaped the history of sugar intake, and the demonization of healthy fats.

Our history is what has caused you to hold this book in your hands. Our hope is that this book becomes a catalyst for your decision to take personal responsibility for yourself and your health. Our hope is to inspire you to become your own advocate for the truth. One word of warning. When you are exposed to the truth, it becomes much harder to ignore or to look the other way. It becomes harder to accept the status quo.

We want you to take charge of your healthcare and to invest in yourself instead of just accepting being told to just take another pill or exercise more. We suggest you form a partnership with medical professionals who are awakening to this history as well. More of them are taking the personal responsibility to become better educated about this history as well. We are grateful to witness this. Many doctors are learning the truth.

We believe and have hope that this personal education by those in the medical community, combined with the moms and grandmothers leading the charge to get better educated on the material in this book, is a great first step and starting place to begin moving in a new and better direction.

All new directions or journeys are started with an idea. The very fact that this book exists started the same way. Two regular guys became friends through common experience and results of the ketogenic lifestyle. Sometimes taking that first step can seem difficult or scary, but once taken, the journey can become exciting. The decision to write this book provided us with this same difficult and scary first step, and we decided just to take that first step and get started, just as we did with our ketogenic journeys.

We are grateful that we took that step, and we encourage you to take in this information. Take your first step to a healthier life and family. We hope that the simple steps we are going to share will get you pointed in the right direction and make that transition much easier. Welcome to the First Steps 2 Keto.

To end this chapter, we would like to share the story of a woman we have worked with. Shalee Green is the mother of three beautiful children and lives in Florida, and here is her story:

## SHALEE'S STORY

"You have type 2 diabetes," the doctor said.

The words shook her to the core. Shalee had struggled with her weight all of her life. She had also lost loved ones to diabetes and poor health due to alcoholism and smoking. She knew she didn't want to end up like that.

In September of 2018 she gave birth to her twins. Although this was an amazingly happy time, Shalee tipped the scales at her all-time heaviest weight. She felt like she had tried every diet under the sun and literally didn't know what to do. Then she saw the post on social media made by a friend who had lost 50 pounds and looked great. She learned about the ketogenic lifestyle and found Ian's keto group.

From there she heard about a 30-Day Challenge that Ian and Jim decided to do that was teaching everything she was wanting to learn to get started the right way. Shalee made the decision to learn about a supplement called Smart Coffee and dove head first into the first challenge.

Shalee is now 42 pounds lighter and no longer type 2 diabetic. She loves the new lifestyle she is living so much that she continues to support new members of the challenge group as an admin. She has found that sharing what she has learned with others is the best kind of help she can get for herself. Thanks to First Steps 2 Keto she has finally started learning what does and does not work for her body. Most important, she has realized it is her responsibility to teach her three children better from the start!

# CHAPTER 3

# Some Simple Steps to Implement the Ketogenic Lifestyle

Now that we have provided some background information, so you know more about us and our experience on a personal level, let's talk about some of the simple steps to transition into the ketogenic lifestyle.

Ian ultimately got his health back by hiring a coach, paying lots of money for training sessions and meal plans, and just doing what he was told. Ian was busy just like you may be. He worked in the chemical industry for 25 years on rotating 12-hour shifts and averaging one day off per month the final 10 years of employment. A schedule like this involved going to bed at 10-11pm and getting up on work days at 3am. Working nights meant getting into bed at 6-7am and sleeping until noon. Ian did not cook, and drive-through windows were the option of choice. It was convenient.

Although being busy is a reality for many of us, it can also be a convenient excuse not to take personal responsibility. When Ian hired his coach, the coach insisted that Ian start cooking for himself and meal prepping to be prepared every single day.

A part of being prepared meant making some changes. The first of these changes was really important. The coach made a simple request: clean the garbage out of your cabinets. If the bad food is not in your house, it is much more difficult to eat. This step makes things easier on yourself when getting started. This simple step, all these years later, is still a powerful step. It can be difficult at first, especially if there are other people in the house that aren't choosing the ketogenic lifestyle. If this is your situation, segregate your ketogenic food if possible. Have your own safe place, such as your own "keto cabinet."

*Everyone is different.* You will see and hear us preach this repeatedly through this book. If you are a single person, your pressures and considerations will be different from a couple who live together. The couple who live together will have different considerations from those with children in the house who have their own eating preferences. There is a universal truth in that all of us have to take personal responsibility for ourselves first before we can be an example to others.

From our experience, leading others into a healthier lifestyle comes from setting the example. We cannot force others to make this decision, and this can be challenging when others close to us in our lives choose not to join us. We cannot give you what advice it will take for you to be successful other than to say this: Your decision is about YOU. Ultimately, this is about you, taking personal responsibility for you, and your health and wellness. If other adults in your life choose to join you, it is their choice.

You are ultimately responsible for your children and the food they put in their body. We believe that moms and dads will have to come to a place in their keto journey and education that concerns what you allow your children to eat. This is an entirely different challenge that we have seen many times now. While some parents have a much easier transition with kids, some have a battle. We can only suggest that getting connected to others who have been through this same situation can be a powerful source of strength.

That is what is most important. If you do not develop this mindset and make this personal decision, you cannot lead anyone else if you cannot lead yourself. Nobody likes a know-it-all, either. Keep quiet and let your results make the noise. This attracts others to want to know what you are doing. We strongly suggest finding a group that is on the same journey as you, led by someone with experience in making this transition.

Years later, the original simple step I learned from my coach has been slightly modified:

## Step One in First Steps 2 Keto is:

### Clean out the garbage!!

We are not asking you to waste food. Feel free to donate it to charity. Getting it out of your house is what is important. You may also consider rearranging things if you have a partner or children that will continue to eat food that is not ketogenic. Consider your own safe space in the pantry or cabinets where you don't have to see those foods that trigger cravings. Have a plan to exchange out some of these things with keto friendly snacks.

To whatever extent possible in your particular situation, get carbs and sugar out of your house and replace with the staples of the ketogenic lifestyle. This may seem overwhelming at first, but this is a hack to make learning about foods easier: *search engines are your friend.*

You now have access to more information with a smartphone or computer with internet access than at any time in human history. Search whatever the food is followed by nutrition label or ingredients. This is something you will start putting into practice, so why not start now?

Specifically look at the **carbs.** You will also get better educated on reading labels and the 56 different names the USA government allows to be used for sugar.

# SUGAR

Buttered Sugar Cane Sugar Dextrose **Caramel**
**Brown Sugar** Corn
Syrup Cane Juice Corn Syrup Solids
Beet Sugar
Confectioner's Sugar Dehydrated Galactose
**Agave** **Demerara Sugar** Cane Juice **Fruit Juice**
**Nectar**
Maltodextrin **Diastatic Malt** **Concentrate**
**Fructose** Diatase
Malt Mannitol Florida Molasses Maltose
Carob Sugar **Sorghum** Crystals
Syrup **Syrup** Treacle Sorbitol Yellow
Sugar
Syrup Sucrose Panocha Raw **Rice Syrup**
**Lactose** Sugar
Castor Sugar Muscovado
HFCS (High Fructose Golden
Barbados Sugar Corn Syrup) Sugar **Glocose Solids**
**Barley Malt** Grape Sugar Mayple Syrup Honey
**Refiner's Syrup** Sugar (granulated) Turbinado
Golden Syrup **Fruit Juice** Sugar
Glucose Date Sugar Icing Sugar
Ethyl Maltol **Dextron**

Carbs = sugar and sugar is the root cause of obesity, heart disease and diabetes. Most of us getting started will aim for around 20 grams of carbs *per day*, but as you start paying attention, you will find you have been consuming this many carbs *per serving* of different foods in multiple meals per day.

Combine that with sodas, snacks, ice cream treats, and what we consume at drive-through windows and it's easy to see the reason we are getting so unhealthy and overweight. Most people simply pay no attention and just eat something when hungry. Many of these fast foods today are scientifically created to bypass the feedback loop to the brain that tells the brain we are not hungry.

This sounds crazy, but it is true.

For those reading this book with children or partners that are not eating ketogenic, we cannot give you a perfect answer for all situations. This will require communication and compromise and a willingness to work it out together. We are not attempting to solve every different problem or circumstance you may have. This is another good reason to belong to a group of people on the same journey together.

Something we all have to learn is that your body does not know the difference between different types or names for sugar. It only knows and responds to the increase in blood glucose caused by the food and drinks we choose to ingest. The pancreas responds by secreting the hormone insulin into the bloodstream to get our blood sugar back down to "normal." Insulin works with glucose to shuttle it into the cells of the body to create energy.

It is one issue to clean out foods that are not ketogenic and another issue to replace these things with staples of the ketogenic lifestyle. Most people just getting started have no idea what ketogenic staples are. We propose the following as a good starting point. This will be a work in progress.

Consider adding a few items per week and marking them off the list or adding items as a meal plan or recipe calls for them. Mapping out a week's worth of meals can make this an easier challenge to conquer instead of dealing with one recipe or meal at a time.

## Ketogenic staples

### Ketogenic Foods: Meats and Cheese

| MEATS | | CHEESES | |
|---|---|---|---|
| Ribeye | Pork Steak | Cheddar | Feta |
| Sirloin | Pork Chops | Mozzarella | Cream Cheese |
| T-Bone | Pork Roast | Parmesan | Mascarpone |
| Chuck Roast | Fish (fatty is best) | Swiss | Goat Cheese |
| Filet Mignon | Shellfish | Colby | Gouda |
| Ground Beef | Sausage | Brie | Blue Cheese |
| Poultry | Bacon | Asiago | Provolone |

NOTE: Leaner poultry meats like chicken and turkey with skin on will increase fats and is great! Alternatively, add some coconut oil, butter, etc. to increase fats if needed. Cheese should be full fat.

### Ketogenic Foods: Refrigerator, Pantry and Other

| REFRIGERATOR, PANTRY AND OTHER | | | |
|---|---|---|---|
| Eggs | Almond Flour | Extracts (vanilla, etc.) | Seasonings |
| Bone Broth | Coconut Flour | Stevia | Xanthan Gum |
| Almond Milk | Coconut Flakes | Swerve Granular | Gelatin |
| Coffee | Quest multipurpose | Swerve Confectioners | Baking Powder |
| Pickles | Pork Rinds | Truvia | Cocoa powder |
| Coconut Cream | Sour Cream | Torani Syrups | Nuts / Nut butter |
| Lily's Chocolate | Sugar Free Ketchup | Walden Farms Syrups | Mustard |

NOTE: Torani has sugar free syrups (BLUE label, NOT the red label). Walden Farms syrups are all sugar free and calorie free. Lily's chocolate is in bars or chips (get no sugar added). Watch carbs in nuts!

We are finding that more grocery stores are carrying these keto staples. If your local grocer does not, consider asking to speak to a manager and ask them to stock an item that you need. Many of them are more than willing to do so. Or simply order online and have the products delivered to your home. Acquiring these ketogenic staples is simply a challenge to overcome.

## Ketogenic Foods: Fats and Vegetables

| FATS | | VEGETABLES | |
|------|------|------|------|
| Butter | Cacao Butter | Avocado | Mushrooms |
| Ghee | Half and Half | Romaine Lettuce | Zucchini |
| Heavy Whipping Cream | MCT Oil | Spinach | Summer Squash |
| Coconut Oil | Mayonnaise | Arugula | Cabbage |
| Avocado oil | Coconut Cream | Swiss Chard | Asparagus |
| Macadamia Oil | Tallow | Celery | Cauliflower |
| Olive Oil | Lard | Bok Choy | Tomato |

NOTE: Fats can also come from fattier cuts of meat like marbled ribeye, fatty fish and even eggs or whole avocado. Add butter to vegetables to increase fats (vegetables are a vessel for butter).

Please do not consider this list anywhere close to complete. This is a simple list of some staples just to give an idea of some of the foods we stock up on.

We are a huge fan of keto friendly seasonings and for those who join us in our 30-Day Challenge, we will share all of our favorites and personal choices with the First Steps 2 Keto Challenge Crew.

# Step 2 in First Steps 2 Keto is:

*Become open-minded to learn*

## What is ketogenic eating?

The ketogenic way of eating is figuring out the total calories per day a person needs to eat to maintain their current weight in the proper ratios of protein, fat and carbs. This is what we call figuring personal macros.

Some people dive in head first and just cut the carbs they eat back to 5-10% of total daily calories. Most people make the simple goal of keeping the total grams of carbs at 20 grams per day or less.

We have also experienced people start off with 50 grams per day of carbs and still get weight loss results. They have the option of slowly cutting back the carbs in a measured amount per day over time, while slowly stair-stepping the healthy fat consumed up over time. This allows for more of an easing into the ketogenic lifestyle as opposed to going all in immediately from the start. It is less shocking to the body and allows for adaptation to less carbs and more healthy fats over time. This can give the digestive system some time to adapt to a higher healthier fat content in the foods we eat.

Neither way is right or wrong. It is just different paths that lead to the same place. One path may have more difficult immediate consequences of keto flu or digestive issues while getting used to more fat being consumed, while the other may not offer results as fast but may do a better job of minimizing or eliminating some of the side effects of getting started in this new way of eating.

The only way to really know if you are staying close to the proper personal macro ratios of ketogenic eating is to track the actual foods eaten each day. There are many apps available that make tracking food and calculating and displaying the ratios of calories of the foods we eat simple. We also work with those in our 30-Day Challenge to get the app you choose set up properly.

The apps or websites can seem complicated at first. Once again, this is just practice and learning new things. For every app there are tutorial videos and videos made by users that walk us through how to use the app to enter foods at meals, to add entire recipes, and even how to use the camera on a smartphone to zap in the UPC code to automatically input all the nutrition information. Tracking becomes much easier over time with practice.

The only other option is guessing. From our experience, we have seen a few people get lucky. They cut their carbs back and add some healthy fats but don't track anything and get results. This person is definitely an exception and we don't recommend this approach.

We suggest just making a decision to get started that best suits YOU and your personality. Whatever way it is that you choose, follow the other steps in this book to be prepared for the possibility of keto flu by having a good electrolyte on hand, having a month's supply of exogenous ketones, and having a stock of bone broth to use. All of these supplements can contribute to minimizing or eliminating many of the negative side effects of getting off the sugar roller coaster.

Some naysayers will always be there to point out that they did not use these supplements when they started the ketogenic lifestyle. They did it without all that and did just fine. We say good for them for doing it the hardest possible way. We don't see them driving around in a horse and buggy even though the automobile has been invented. Do they shun air travel just because their ancestors never flew on a plane? Do they still have a rotary phone at home, or are they now attached to a smartphone like the vast majority of humanity? People are interesting in this way.

Technology continues to evolve and while some people may feel like starting the ketogenic lifestyle is very complicated, these advances in technology have actually made things much easier for the new person to get started as well as have much better success at sustaining this lifestyle.

We do agree that many companies have jumped on the keto bandwagon and are putting the word keto on anything just to sell it. There are definitely some garbage products out in the marketplace that don't offer any measurable benefit, and more are being pushed out all the time.

There is no way to do a comprehensive review of every product and supplement out there, but we will share some insight on things we have personally used and tested with measurable benefits and the backing of time, experience and science.

Those products we do recommend are based on personal testing and repeated results and benefits received with the vast majority of people that we have recommended these products to. Only when these results show this repeatability are we willing to recommend them. For some products, there are many options to test or purchase from. We also have very specific reasons for what we recommend to others. Some of these reasons include transparency in labeling, ingredient sourcing, price, and some are just based on amazing results.

Each of us is different and will have to make the personal choice of investing in things that we recommend that makes the transition into the ketogenic lifestyle easier and more sustainable.

Each of us has a personal decision to spend the money to minimize a possible negative side effect, or to invest in something that may provide a much more positive result.

Things like bone broth have so many positive benefits. Exogenous ketones and electrolytes are an option for dealing with symptoms of keto flu. Another new technology we have been recommending and seeing great results with is Smart Coffee.

Many people already drink coffee or a hot or cold chocolate beverage and add healthy fats to boost the fat content up. The technology has now been created utilizing coffee or chocolate as a delivery system for all-natural ingredients that curb hunger and cravings (powerful for implementing intermittent fasting), while effecting release of the pleasure and reward chemicals of the brain (just as comfort food does).

We have experienced great results and demonstrated the fact that when our mood is elevated, we do better at all things in life. Getting a boost of clean energy as well as mental focus and clarity during a lifestyle change is very beneficial to a more positive result.

Different people, coaches, or groups may have their own supplements or products that are recommended based on their own personal experience and results. It will be your personal choice to do your own test to determine if these products benefit you. Again, there will be those who point out they didn't use any of these supplements, and we will readily agree they are not for everyone and may not be for you. We promote allowing people to make the choice for themselves. Please don't rob another person of their chance at success based on your personal choice. Allow others the respect to make their own choices. Don't be the reason someone failed because of your opinion.

# Step 3 in First Steps 2 Keto is:

## *Figure your personal macros*

Although this topic is confusing to many new people, we want to do our best to provide this simple definition. Macros stands for macronutrients. This consists of the protein, fats and carbohydrates we consume every day. Most people simply have no idea how many calories they consume each day, much less understand what ratios of fats, protein and carbs make up their daily food intake.

Every human being has a total number of calories that they can consume on a daily basis that, based on their current personal situation and statistics, would not cause them to lose or gain weight. This is not magic. It is science. If a human utilizes the same total of calories for energy as they consume when eating, then their body weight should remain the same.

We refer to this as *maintenance calories*. If a person eats more calories than they burn with activity, they will gain weight, and a person will lose weight if they have a calorie deficit of food compared to energy burned from activity. This is all very straightforward so far, but let's discuss the variables that affect personal macro calculations. Gender, age, height, activity level and current body weight all affect the calculations.

This is why one person comparing their personal macros to someone else is a waste of time. *We are all different.* What is important is knowing our personal macros. The simple definition of the ketogenic way of eating is consuming the daily macros in certain ratios. Ketogenic eating is a higher healthy fat, moderate protein and low-carb way of eating. When we look at the ratio of macros consumed on a daily basis, a fairly standard keto ratio is 70% fat, 25% protein and 5% carbohydrate.

Considering that the majority of humans simply eat when hungry (or when they are "supposed to eat") and continue to eat until "full," most people simply have no idea how many calories they consume or what ratio of their daily calories consists of fats, protein and carbs.

Let's go ahead and address the fact that in the realm of ketogenic eating there are opinions that range from one extreme (lazy keto) to the other (hard core keto). Some people have some very extremist views on what is or isn't considered "keto." They may look at individual foods and declare them "not keto." Some of this is the repeating of what they were taught. Some people have severe medical challenges such as brain or some other serious cancer that may cause them to be much stricter than an otherwise healthy person just looking to drop a few pounds to look better in their swimsuit for vacation.

For the purposes of this book, focused on the newest person just getting started, we decided to take the middle ground. Once again, we will state that everyone is different and is on their own journey. We will not promote any extreme of the spectrum of what is considered ketogenic eating and simply state that you will have plenty of time to decide where you fit into the ketogenic lifestyle. We suggest you base it on *results* and not on what some keto guru thinks.

The truth is that we all have personal macros. A tiny person's total maintenance calories will be less than a larger person. For the sake of this discussion, let's pick an average maintenance calorie number for "Bob."

If Bob consumes food each day and the total calories equals 2000, he will neither gain nor lose weight. Bob could decide to keep eating the way he always has but cut his daily intake of calories by 500 calories per day *(calorie deficit)*. Seven days, times a 500-calorie deficit per day, equals 3500 calories in a week; 3500 calories would be the calories in one pound of fat. Therefore, if Bob only consumes 1500 calories per day, he should lose an average of one pound per week. If Bob eats more than 2000 calories per day, he will be in a *calorie surplus* and start to steadily gain weight as time goes on.

Macros are made up of calories. Protein and carbs contain four calories per gram while fat contains nine calories per gram. Yes, fat contains slightly more than twice the calories of protein or carbs.

A common mistake new people make is trying to ratio the *grams* of macros they are eating instead of the *total calories* per day they are eating. Because dietary fat is twice the calories as protein and carbs, this causes the math to be incorrect. Let's examine it the correct way.

Bob decides to do the ketogenic way of eating. His maintenance calories are 2000 calories per day. Bob doesn't want to lose weight but is seeking other health benefits. After doing a little research, Bob uses a macro calculator to input his personal information. Bob has seen all kinds of ratios for the ketogenic way of eating but decides to start slowly and sets his fat ratio at 65%. 2000 calories times 65% equals 1300 calories a day from fat.

Bob chooses 25% as his ratio for protein. 2000 calories times 25% equals 500 calories from protein. This leaves 10% for carbs. 2000 times 10% equals 200 calories from carbs.

*1300 calories from fat divided by nine calories per gram = 144 grams of fat for the day.

*500 calories from protein divided by four calories per gram equals 125 grams of protein.

*200 calories from carbs divided by four calories per gram equals 50 grams of carbs.

While some people can make progress eating 50 grams of carbs per day, many others must be stricter, and a common rule of thumb is to target only 20 grams per day of carbs. 20 grams times four calories per gram is only 80 calories per day. The simple thing is to select an app such as MyFitnessPal or Carb Manager and input your personal info and weight loss goal, and the app will do the calculations for you. We do not recommend setting the weight loss goal for more than one pound per week/four pounds per month.

One suggestion that we make is that if you have extra body fat you want to burn off, consider starting at a lower ratio of fat like 60-65% and a slightly higher ratio of protein while keeping carbs lower. This allows the body to get used to the higher fat content, and now the person is utilizing body fat for fuel, as well as slightly higher fat in food consumed. Some apps give you the ability to change these ratios.

As body fat content comes down, simply bump up the fat ratio in the app about 5% per month until reaching your ideal ratios. Most people that do this find an easier transition to a higher fat content in what they eat.

There is absolutely nothing wrong with this approach of easing into the ketogenic lifestyle. Other people prefer to just set the ratios at 70% fat, 25% protein, and 5% carbs from the start and just go for it. The point is that you have options on how you want to get started in the ketogenic way of eating.

# Step 4 in First Steps 2 Keto is:

## Implementing ketogenic eating

Many people have heard about keto. These people may have family, friends, or coworkers who have had some measure of success by changing the way they eat. When these people decide to implement the ketogenic way of eating, they are overwhelmed with many ideas and opinions of how to start.

They just want to know what to do to get going. This is one of the major reasons we decided to write a book like this. We want to support people in getting started right.

First Steps 2 Keto is a concept born out of the fact that when we looked around, we found some very limited information that we felt did not cover enough detail on subjects we consider really important, or provided so much information as to be overwhelming. There are also now so many opinions in the keto space, from one extreme to the other, that it is difficult to know who to listen to.

We feel that we are positioned firmly in the middle of these extremes. Ultimately it will be you, who we consistently suggest becoming your own best advocate, to take responsibility and do some personal research and to make a personal decision about who you will choose to follow and why. We fully realize that everyone is on their own journey. We of course would love you to get started and stay connected to us, but our honest hope is to get you started on your own personal journey of better health and wellness. We want to provide some sound but simple steps and guidelines to move you forward into a sustainable lifestyle. This requires good information from the start.

Many people just start cutting carbs and jump on the keto bandwagon without any understanding of why they are cutting the carbs, what ketogenic eating actually is, and what will happen in and to their body when they make this choice. The book you are reading will provide this information. We believe it can be really important to take a look at the actual food being eaten before making any changes.

Taking a look at the total calories being consumed each day and the ratios of carb, protein and fats will paint a realistic picture of the way we have been eating in contrast to the difference in changing to the ketogenic way of eating.

The Standard American Diet is 50% carbohydrate. This is *sugar* or foods that break down quickly and turn into glucose inside the body. These consumed carbs increase the blood glucose level and create an insulin response from the pancreas. The pancreas and the insulin that is added to the bloodstream have the job of bringing glucose levels back down to a "normal" level by working together to shuttle the glucose from the bloodstream and into the cells of the body to create energy.

High glucose levels cause problems (diabetes) and low blood glucose levels cause problems (hypoglycemia). We will pause here to state that we have seen and experienced lower blood sugar readings while in a state of ketosis. It is a different experience when the body has a fuel source like ketones available than it is without the presence of an energy source like ketones. This is something each individual person will have to experience and understand how their body responds in situations like this.

Once again, the only way a person will truly know what blood ketone levels and blood glucose levels really are is to test with a meter. We provide a discount link to our preferred meter to all who join us in our First Steps 2 Keto 30-Day Challenge.

We also strongly recommend that anyone starting the ketogenic lifestyle takes a minute to familiarize themselves with the glycemic index. This is a *comparison* of common foods we eat *to table sugar*.

We will not get into the entire list in this book, but hopefully sharing a few examples of common foods compared to sugar will help you understand how blood glucose is affected by eating these foods. Our body does not understand the difference in ingesting table sugar added to food or eating a piece of fruit. Our body only responds to the effect on our blood sugar increasing.

Sugar is given a score of 100 on the glycemic index, and other foods are given a numeric value based on how they affect blood glucose when ingested and generally fall into a low, medium or high glycemic index category. The following foods fall into the *high* glycemic index category and a few in the *medium* category:

Once again this is a limited list just for quick reference. Please take a look at the entire glycemic index and bookmark it in your device as a quick reference tool.

| | | |
|---|---|---|
| Dates 100 | French fries 76 | Brown rice 72 |
| French bread 97 | Cereals 76 | Tapioca 70 |
| White rice 91 | Doughnuts 75 | Taco shells 68 |
| Baked potato 85 | Soda 74 | Corn meal 68 |
| Cornflakes 84 | Mashed potato 73 | Croissant 67 |
| Mashed potato (instant) 83 | Honey 73 | Bran muffin 65 |
| Rice cakes 82 | Watermelon 72 | Hamburger bun 61 |
| Pretzels 81 | Corn chips 72 | Sourdough 57 |
| White bread 79 | Bagel 72 | Pita, white 57 |

Once again it bears repeating: the body doesn't know the difference between table sugar and these foods. It only knows that when these foods are ingested blood glucose is affected in the same way as ingesting sugar (based on this index). This is important information to understand as ketogenic eating is implemented. If you are unsure about a food, the glycemic index is easy to refer to.

The more we learn to pay attention, read labels, and identify the hidden sugars we didn't even realize were in the foods we eat, the stronger we become at not allowing hidden sugars to affect our ketone levels.

A word on *maltodextrin.* This is an ugly word to get familiar with right away. Maltodextrin is a white powder made from corn, rice, potato starch, or wheat. None of these ingredients is a part of the ketogenic way of eating, and even though it comes from plants, it is highly processed. These starches are cooked and then acids or enzymes such as heat-stable alpha-amylase are added to further break down the starches. The resulting white powder is water-soluble and has a neutral taste.

Although considered safe by the FDA, maltodextrin is even higher on the glycemic index than sugar. If you find enough maltodextrin in something you eat or a product you take, it can spike your blood sugar worse than sugar does. Sugar is 100 on the glycemic index and maltodextrin can range from 106-136. This ingredient is inexpensive to produce, and food companies are putting it into *everything* as a thickening agent and sweetener. Maltodextrin has been shown to have a negative impact on gut bacteria. We recommend you **stay away** from this ingredient. (Healthline)

## Learning what to eat and who to listen to

A common goal for most people is to limit daily carb intake to 20 grams or less. Here are some examples of carb content in common foods most people eat every day, and the following contain approximately **15 grams of carbs per serving:**

## Bread

1 slice white bread toast
$\frac{1}{2}$ small bagel
$\frac{1}{2}$ English muffin
$\frac{1}{2}$ a hotdog or hamburger bun
1 x 5" pancake or waffle
1 x 6" tortilla
1 small muffin

## Cereal

$\frac{1}{2}$ cup bran, granola, or cooked cereal like oats
$\frac{1}{2}$ cup sweetened cereal
$\frac{3}{4}$ cup plain dry cereal
$1\frac{3}{4}$ cup puffed cereal

## Rice, beans, grains, pasta

$\frac{1}{3}$ cup cooked pasta
$\frac{1}{3}$ cup cooked grains
$\frac{1}{3}$ cup baked beans
$\frac{1}{2}$ cup cooked beans
$\frac{1}{2}$ cup corn or green peas
$\frac{1}{2}$ cup cooked potatoes
10-15 French fries
$\frac{1}{2}$ cup spaghetti sauce

## Fruits

1 small apple, orange or pear
$\frac{1}{2}$ banana
$\frac{3}{4}$ cup blueberries or raspberries
$\frac{1}{3}$ of a cantaloupe

1 cup cubed melon
15 cherries
15 grapes
1 ¼ cup strawberries
¾ cup pineapple

## Milk/yogurt

10 oz. skim, 1%, 2%, whole milk
½ cup evaporated milk
⅓ cup dry milk powder
1 cup plain yogurt

## Soups

1 cup broth-based soup with noodles
½ cup bean, split pea, or lentil
1 cup cream-based soup

## Combination foods: approx. 30 grams of carbs

| | |
|---|---|
| 1 cup beef stew | 1 cup ravioli |
| 1 meat burrito | 2 soft tacos |
| 2 stuffed cannelloni | 1 slice of pizza |
| 12 chicken nuggets | ⅔ cup macaroni and cheese |
| 1 cup chili with beans | 3" x 4" piece of lasagna |

This is a sample of some normal foods many people consume, just to get an idea of the carbs we are taking in from these choices. When researching carb content, use a search engine to search for the food along with nutrition labels and *ingredients*. Do this for any food you want to learn about.

You must be your own advocate. Companies are jumping on the keto bandwagon and putting the name keto on every kind of food just to sell it. As mentioned previously, the government allows companies to use 56 different names for sugar on food labels. If you see a product with the word keto on it and it contains maltodextrin or any of the 56 names for sugar, you can be sure the company is just marketing the word and is not serious about your health or the ketogenic lifestyle.

One of the things we regretfully must point out is concerning charities, non-profits, and organizations/associations who claim to have the interest of public health as their first mission and priority. Some of these organizations have amazing volunteers and do a great job of raising a lot of money. Some of these organizations have been around for generations and are totally trusted.

While the average person who looks to these organizations for guidance on health and wellbeing can certainly make a contribution, it doesn't take a financial investigator to follow the money. In the 2011-2012 financial statement, an organization focused on heart health noted $521 million in donations from non-government/non-membership sources; and many well-known large drug companies, including statin producers, contribute in the million-dollar range.

What about all those cereals, full of sugar, with that heart healthy check mark on the box? Moms and grandmothers all across the land keep feeding this "heart healthy" cereal to their children and grandchildren because it has that check mark on the box.

Another interesting event that occurred in 2018 involved the organization suddenly changing their guidelines for what constitutes hypertension. Yes, that means high blood pressure. All of a sudden, from one day to the next, just like magic, 14 million Americans who were totally healthy yesterday now qualify for a statin drug to save them from a heart attack. This doesn't seem like such a bad thing until we get a real look at what the numbers mean.

This image represents the percentage of people actually helped by lowering the blood pressure guidelines. While 14 million people are now being told they need to be on a blood pressure drug, it has to make a reasonable person wonder who is actually benefiting from these guidelines. *Image used with permission and credit to Dr. Andy Lazris and Erik Rifkin.*

Those four people represented by the black dots out of this entire theater of people who are now told their blood pressure is too high may actually benefit. We have to ask who actually benefits from lowering the guidelines?

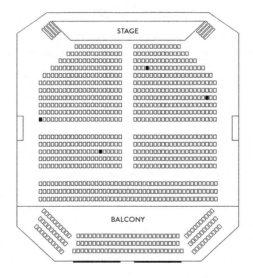

**A theatre aid that shows the number of people helped by a lower blood pressure target in SPRINT. Courtesy of Dr. Andy Lazris and Erik Rifkin**

Finally, we want to point out that this organization stated that coconut oil isn't healthy and never has been, which came from a lead author of the report. As reported in the *USA Today* article, "Coconut oil isn't healthy. It's never been healthy."

"The Dietary Fats and Cardiovascular Disease advisory reviewed existing data on saturated fat, showing coconut oil increased LDL ('bad') cholesterol in seven out of seven controlled trials. Researchers didn't see a difference between coconut oil and other oils high in saturated fat, like butter, beef fat and palm oil. In fact, 82% of the fat in coconut oil is saturated, according to the data – far beyond butter (63%), beef fat (50%) and pork lard (39%).

"Because coconut oil increases LDL cholesterol, a cause of CVD [cardiovascular disease], and has no known offsetting favorable effects, we advise against the use of coconut oil," this association said in the Dietary Fats and Cardiovascular Disease advisory.

In our opinion, as a couple of regular guys who never paid any attention to stuff like this whatsoever, that is a glaring example of a 100% healthy product being demonized by an organization that is supposedly looking out for the public. You don't have to take our word for it. After all, we are just a couple of regular guys who got really sick by following all these guidelines. It wasn't good for us, but it was great for the drug companies.

It is not that difficult to do a little research and see that coconut oil *increases HDL* (good cholesterol) and *increases the particle size of LDL cholesterol* making it bigger and "fluffy" instead of small and sticky.

When it becomes apparent that important details are being overlooked or ignored, seemingly to produce the desired outcome of an establishment instead of the truth, we are merely suggesting that instead of assuming that your health and best interest is being served by any association that takes in multimillion-dollar donations from the food and drug industry you should consider becoming your own best health advocate.

Here is some information on coconut oil from some actual respected doctors who have earned our trust. We are grateful for all we have learned from them.

# Dr. Mark Hyman

Coconut oil is a medium-chain triglyceride (MCT) oil. There are many health benefits from consuming coconut oil, some of which are:

1.   Reduce body fat

2.   Help balance hormones

3.   Control appetite

4.   Lower insulin levels

5.   Strengthen immune system

6.   Tons more...

"Countries with the highest intakes of coconut oil have the lowest rates of heart disease."

"One study among lean, heart disease- and stroke-free Pacific Islanders who consumed up to 63% of their calories from coconut fat found total cholesterol rose but so did their 'good' HDL."

*We must suppose the lead author didn't get the memo about the 'good' cholesterol going up too, or any of the other well-known health benefits that are agreed upon by many amazing and well-known doctors.

# Dr. Stephen Sinatra

## Co-author of *The Great Cholesterol Myth*

Here are just a few of many facts shared by Dr. Sinatra and Dr. Bowden in the book:

*The hypothetical link between high levels of total cholesterol and heart disease has *never* been proven. It is a diagnosis conjured up to serve drug companies who want to sell more cholesterol-lowering statin drugs.

*Cholesterol levels are a poor predictor of heart attacks. Only about 50% of heart attack victims have high cholesterol and 50% of people with high cholesterol do not have heart disease.

*Recent studies suggest statin drugs are associated with a higher risk of diabetes which is a major risk factor for heart disease.

*Dr. Sinatra and Dr. Bowden agree while big pharma is busy raking in over $31 billion annually by selling drugs for high-cholesterol with terrible side effects, to unknowing victims, these companies' financial success is putting the American public's health at risk.

## Dr. Malcolm Kendrick

Dr. Malcolm Kendrick is a co-author of a new study involving nearly 70,000 people, in which he discovered that there was no link between "bad" cholesterol and the premature deaths of over 60-year-olds from cardiovascular disease.

"What we found in our detailed systematic review was that older people with high LDL (low-density lipoprotein) levels, the so-called 'bad' cholesterol, lived longer and had less heart disease." (Steemit. com)

Once again, we share this information with you to prove the point that you must become your own best advocate. YOU are the only one that truly has your best interest at heart, literally, when it comes down to it. We admit that we did not pay any attention to things like this in the past, but once our eyes were opened to different sources of information it becomes impossible to ignore. We feel it is our responsibility to share what we have learned with others.

We truly feel blessed to have experienced all we have, and we want to do our best to shorten the learning curve for others. We both felt totally alone when we started our personal journey. We both remember, vividly, the feeling that we were the only person that we knew that was practicing the ketogenic lifestyle.

Even though we didn't do it perfectly at first, and it has taken continuous practice, failure and getting back up one more time, we feel compelled to share with others what we have learned. The shorter we make the learning curve for those just getting started, the higher the success rate we see of those maintaining this lifestyle.

The next thing we want to share is very useful information to know for those first starting the ketogenic lifestyle: ketosis, ketones and keto flu. Understanding the basics of ketosis, ketones and the keto flu is fundamental to really understanding what the ketogenic lifestyle is about. It is one thing to have heard about keto and to decide to try it for yourself. It is something entirely on another level to understand why you should.

## Step 5 of First Steps 2 Keto is:

### *Understand ketosis and keto flu*

Ketosis is another word that seems to bring out the confusion in people, and for good reason. Dr. Robert Atkins published his low-carb diet book in 1972, and the updated paperback version was published in 2002 as low-carb eating started gaining in popularity.

Ian first learned of the word ketosis in 1995 when he first read this book about low-carb dieting. The Atkins Diet was the very first introduction to the word ketosis. This was true for most people that even knew about low-carb dieting back then. Cutting back on sugar was the only possible way, other than starvation or long-term fasting (that mimics starvation) to achieve this state of ketosis. Most people equated ketosis with utilizing body fat for fuel as a way of losing weight.

Now that the technology of exogenous ketones is available (more on this later), some companies and marketing strategies have used terms like "instant ketosis", and while this is technically correct, simply elevating ketones in the body, it is **not** burning body fat for fuel. This has caused some confusion to those new to the ketogenic lifestyle. Exposure to marketing like this can certainly be confusing.

Let us try to simplify the explanation and help you to better understand. In our opinion, the proper terminology should be ketogenesis. Ketogenesis is the creation of ketones in the liver, by utilizing healthy fats in the diet and stored body fat, released as fatty acids into the bloodstream. This process occurs by choice, based on the foods we choose to eat, by fasting, and due to starvation as a survival mechanism.

By using exogenous (outside the body) ketones, such as BHB ketone salts, a person can elevate the level of ketones in the body, as measured by a blood ketone meter, simply by drinking them in. While this does boost the level of this energy source, this is not the same thing as the body releasing stored fat into the bloodstream, processing it in the liver, and *creating* ketones for energy.

The ketogenesis process of converting stored body fat or dietary fat consumed in meals creates three different measurable types of ketone bodies. The synthesis of these ketone bodies is simply the process of processing and converting fatty acids into a usable source of fuel. Ketones are this fuel source.

## What is a ketone?

The three different ketone bodies produced by the process of converting fatty acids into usable fuel are Acetoacetate, Acetone, and BHB (Beta-hydroxybutyrate). BHB is the most abundant of these ketone bodies followed by Acetoacetate and Acetone.

When blood glucose is low, as it normally was before the proliferation of sugar consumption, the brain gets about 60-70% of its required energy from ketones. The other small amount of glucose required can be created by the human body from other sources in a process called gluconeogenesis. Despite any disinformation suggesting otherwise, the body can create the small amount of glucose it may need from sources other than carbohydrate.

## Understanding keto flu

In 1995, Ian read Dr. Atkins' book and made the decision one day to cut out carbs and "do the Atkins Diet." Within the first couple of days, not only was he experiencing cravings and the symptoms of withdrawal from sugar, but Ian started feeling horrible. He began experiencing nausea, headache, body aches, and other symptoms very similar to having the actual flu. It was so bad he literally almost stopped the low-carb diet just to feel better. Why would anyone put themselves through feeling this way for any reason?

As a matter of fact, having practiced this lifestyle for years now, in addition to the powerful addiction to sugar and the associated science and research food companies invest into marketing foods so we automatically crave more, the symptoms of keto flu is the single reason why most people fail the ketogenic lifestyle.

What Ian didn't know at the time when he first started low-carb eating is that cutting out carbs, in the way that he did, forced his body to start creating ketones for energy. Ian also didn't realize that for every gram of carbs we eat, our bodies will store 3-4 grams of water.

The process of creating ketones is not like flipping a switch. It is a *process* that can take some time, especially when that person has been a glucose burner for decades. The releasing of the stored water weight happens much faster than the creation of ketones. The buildup of ketones in the blood to measurable levels can take days, or longer, for some people to have this energy source available.

We have all heard stories of people or friends who decided to do a low-carb diet and got crazy fast weight loss results. The reality is these crazy fast results are mostly water weight releasing. The good news is that some people drop a lot of water weight quickly. The bad news is that if they start eating carbs again, they will put it back on just as fast. A side effect of this rapid water loss is *electrolyte imbalance.*

This electrolyte imbalance, combined with the total lack of an energy source (glucose or ketones), is what causes people to feel so bad. Combine this condition with withdrawal symptoms, such as cravings for sugar, and this is referred to as *keto flu.* Electrolytes are essential for human health and there is a balance of these nutrients in the body.

Calcium, sodium, magnesium, chloride, potassium and phosphate all aid numerous bodily functions such as muscle function, blood pressure regulation, blood clotting, maintaining fluids of the body, healthy bones and teeth, nerve signaling, and even heartbeat regulation all require electrolytes.

Electrolyte imbalance can occur from excessive sweating and dehydration due to exercise or working outside in hot weather. Understanding this makes it also easy to understand how a rapid change in the amount of water weight we carry can have the same disruptive effect on the balance of electrolytes in the body.

When we make the choice to become a fat burner, it can take days, or longer, for some people to start the process of creating ketones in the body and build up the levels in the blood to start reading on a meter. Anything above .5 mmol on a meter is an indication of ketosis.

For many new people making the decision to start the ketogenic lifestyle, it is exciting to know that you are actually creating ketones in the body. Urine strips were once the testing method of choice, and for those first getting started, this is the only method many people are familiar with.

Aside from the novelty of seeing the urine strip change color, indicating that ketones are present in the urine, we have found that this is not our preferred method to test.

# Step 6 of First Steps 2 Keto is:

### Testing for ketones

Most people I personally know that "did the Atkins Diet" never read the book. They just decided to "cut carbs" and eat lots of meat. They did not seek better education about what was going to happen to them on a low-carb diet. They just decided they were going to "do the Atkins Diet."

Knowing what we know now, we want to provide better education to those who are taking personal responsibility to begin the ketogenic lifestyle. In the past, many people just started eating lots of bacon and eggs, cut out bread, pasta and potatoes, bought some keto-stix (urine test strips) and hoped they turned purple to show they were "in ketosis." Interestingly, many people starting the ketogenic lifestyle today do the exact same thing.

We can share with you now that after years of extensive testing with blood ketone meters, what we have found is that these urine strips, and the associated color chart (ranging from beige to light pink to dark purple), actually provides very little useful information other than the novelty of knowing you have ketones in your body when getting started. These strips only inform you that you are expelling some ketones in your urine. The good news is you are producing some ketones in your body. The bad news is you have no idea what your blood levels are, and blood levels are what is really important.

We have witnessed a blood ketone meter show very little change at all, while the urine strips run from one end of the spectrum to the other: light ketosis to heavy. We have also witnessed the unwarranted and useless stress this has put on every person who has ever used these strips when getting started. New people getting started will equate light pink to "losing" and dark purple to "winning." This is actually not correct as all the color really means is you are expelling more ketones when darker purple. We have seen that as people become better "keto adapted," they will better utilize the ketones for fuel instead of expelling them in urine.

We have experienced people who have probably never had elevated ketones in the body since they were a baby (on mother's milk, full of healthy fats and ketones) start a low-carb way of eating with expectations of immediate results. This is a fundamental failure to understand that the process of adaptation to utilize fat for fuel is a *process*.

It is exactly as we are designed as humans, but after spending decades as a glucose burner as the primary fuel source, it would stand to reason we may have to allow some time to get better adapted to using ketones for fuel. In the meantime, while this adaptation is improving, the non-keto adapted person pees out more ketones not used for energy. We do not store ketones the way we store body fat. We excrete what the body doesn't use for energy. Because of this, we are of the opinion that using a blood ketone/glucose meter is the best way to test for ketones in the body.

Although there are now some breath meters showing up on the market, what we have seen from our personal testing and observation in comparison testing is that the breath meter will demonstrate three readings:

1. **Not in ketosis** (correlates with blood meter)

2. **In ketosis** (correlates with blood meter)

3. **In deep ketosis** (whatever that means, as did not correlate with blood meter)

In our personal testing, as with the urine strips, the breath meter we tested gave no definitive ranges when compared to blood meter readings at "deep ketosis" levels.

Maybe this technology will improve in time, but our opinion, based on years of experience, is that a blood meter is currently the most accurate and reliable way to test the level of ketones circulating in the bloodstream. This is the actual ketone reading of what ketones are available in the bloodstream to be used to create energy, not what is being expelled in breath or urine.

Ketosis is very simply an elevated level of ketones in the body, and by choosing the ketogenic way of eating we force our bodies to utilize fat for fuel. The human body is totally capable of producing the small amount of carbohydrates needed to fuel the systems that require them. This is called gluconeogenesis. That is why you have never heard the term *essential carbohydrate*. There are obviously some essential nutrients we can only get from food or supplementation, but carbohydrates do not apply.

This elevated level of ketones in the body also indicates that an *energy source* is now present. Ketones go into the cells of the body and create energy like glucose does. Ketones actually are the preferred fuel source, when available, and do not require insulin to get into the cells like glucose does. Ketones create almost 40% more energy than glucose per unit of oxygen. The brain will get 60-70% of its energy from ketones, and the body can create the small amount of glucose that makes up the rest.

Despite any myths and misinformation you may hear (and we have heard it all and continue to hear some amazingly wrong and inaccurate things repeated over and over by the media, the medical field, the fitness industry, big pharma, and associations dealing with diabetes), we see with our own eyes that those we work with are able to reduce, minimize and eliminate medications and become the healthiest versions of themselves they have ever been. There is no such thing as an essential carbohydrate.

In the last few years, the technology of exogenous ketones has been brought to the market. While the technology and the product have been misunderstood as people began to experience this new technology, we now have three plus years of personal experience using exogenous ketones and recommending their use to those starting and maintaining the ketogenic lifestyle. The ability to drink ketones into the body (exogenous = from outside) and elevate the level inside the body (endogenous) has been a game-changer for those who previously suffered the keto flu.

The combination of electrolyte imbalance and the lack of an energy source, while glucose stores in the body rapidly deplete while waiting for ketogenesis to build up ketones as the new energy source, can cause a person to feel horrible. Many people are just not willing to endure feeling like this when their sugar-addicted mind is screaming at them to just eat some carbs.

As difficult as it can be to transition to the ketogenic lifestyle, dealing with the symptoms of keto flu can make it even more difficult. Today there are options.

Jim is an example of someone who used exogenous ketones immediately when starting the ketogenic lifestyle. Combining exogenous ketones with supplemental electrolytes allowed Jim to transition from a very unhealthy type 2 diabetic glucose burner to a keto adapted fat burner without suffering **any** effects of keto flu.

When exogenous ketones hit the market, Ian was a partner in a gym. One of the trainers showed him a baggie containing a white powder. It actually looked like something out of the movie *Scar Face*. Ian asked him what the heck was in the baggie and was told "ketones."

"What do you do with it?" Ian asked.

"You drink it," said the trainer.

"Whoever told you that story is seriously misinformed," Ian told the trainer.

It was actually Ian that was misinformed because the technology of exogenous ketones is here, and it is real. The ability to drink the energy source into the body, while the endogenous (inside the body) production process gets started, has shown to be an amazing option. The ability to test with a blood meter and see this increase in blood ketones has been a game-changer for those now making the transition to the ketogenic lifestyle.

Ian became his own test subject and experimented over the next couple of months with different types of diets. The more he tested the product, the more intrigued he became. One thing Ian knew for sure was that he felt fantastically energized using ketones, but the final test came down to going full ketogenic.

Memories of how terrible the keto flu symptoms were that he experienced before came flooding back. Ian was thinking back about how many people had failed before because they simply were not willing to go through the symptoms of keto flu again. Could this really be a solution?

As Ian cut the carbohydrates to a minimum, he just kept drinking the ketones and added in some electrolytes because he had learned about dropping water weight and disrupting electrolyte balance from bodybuilders prepping for shows.

The combination of the two supplements worked almost like magic! As horrible as the symptoms of keto flu had been originally, the keto flu was basically eliminated this time. No headaches or body aches occurred. No feelings of being tired or run down happened either. In fact, the experience was quite the opposite. Using exogenous ketones was literally drinking the energy source that was missing into the body, while waiting for endogenous ketone production to begin and build up to measurable levels in the blood. This was a game-changer.

Just as Jim experienced zero symptoms of keto flu as he started his journey by using exogenous ketones and an electrolyte supplement, Ian was able to duplicate that experience as well. We have shared this simple solution with many people getting started with the ketogenic lifestyle and have minimized or eliminated horrible keto flu symptoms for these people.

We realize that everyone is different. If you don't experience the symptoms of the keto flu, that is awesome for you. If you are one of us that do, these supplements are worth their weight in gold. We recommend this to the newest person getting started. Having a supply of these supplements on hand, if at all possible, is a strong recommendation but not a requirement. If you get a terrible headache or body aches, you always have the option to just tough it out.

If you had a solution available that can minimize or eliminate the negative side effects of keto flu, why in the world would you just tough it out?

# Step 7 in First Steps 2 Keto is:

## *Supplements and ketogenic eating*

One of the arguments against ketogenic eating involves *micronutrients.* Claims have been made that the ketogenic way of eating is not healthy because those who practice it don't get enough vitamins, minerals and other micronutrients. It is easy enough to purchase some multivitamins or multimineral product, but we wanted to make you aware that companies that sell these supposedly healthy supplements have also been adding ingredients like sugar and maltodextrin to their products. *Always read the labels.*

It can be extremely frustrating to begin this new way of life, to cut back on carbs and sugar, and to start testing for blood ketones only to realize that something is keeping us from elevating blood ketone levels. It is especially frustrating when we realize it is because of ingredients added to supposedly healthy supplements or foods that a company is marketing as "keto" or "keto friendly" that upon closer examination are found to contain levels of ingredients like maltodextrin that affect the ability for the body to even get into ketosis.

There are good products available that do not affect ketogenesis at all. It is up to each of us to become diligent at actually reading labels, not making assumptions, and to realize that the word keto has become a marketing ploy just to sell more products. Once again, the only way to actually know for sure how you are personally affected by a food or ingredient, such as sugar alcohols, is to test before and after with a blood meter. We are always on the lookout for products that fit into this lifestyle that contain quality ingredients. We do our best with our groups to educate our members on the difference.

Having previously owned a gym and provided meal plans to the gym members and clients, Ian has been a huge skeptic of the supplement industry in general. Now with years of experience personally using and recommending different supplements and products that he has found that actually work and provide a positive result and benefit, Ian once again points out that everyone is different.

There are good products available, and there are some that we would suggest are not worth the money or that do not provide a measurable result. The only way to know is to do your own personal test. Because something works for one person doesn't mean it will work for every person. Some of us have very individualized issues that must be addressed and improved or overcome that others don't have to consider.

Some supplements available on the market offer no immediate effects on the user. We have to do our research and trust that what the available literature says is the truth. We have to trust that the ingredients and quantities shown on labels are true. We also have to trust that government agencies responsible for oversight of industries like supplements actually do anything to keep bad actors from bringing bad products to market.

The supplement industry does have regulations and guidelines it must follow, but the reality is that supplements are not drugs. They are not regulated in the same way that drugs are, do not have the same requirements or scrutiny that drugs do, and even the agencies of the world that approves drugs doesn't have a perfect track record.

In our experience, we have found some things that we personally have received results and benefits from. We have also tried and tested many things that did not offer any tangible benefit we could point to. We have also seen some marketing campaigns that simply capitalize on the growing popularity of the ketogenic way of eating that seem to target those who lack any experience to know better, and that also target people who want fast results that really are not reasonable.

For the purpose of this book, we will point to the supplement product exogenous ketones pills. When exogenous ketones first came to market, people were paying about $5 per serving for a product that did not provide any quantity of ketone salts on the label. As more companies entered the marketplace, some of them started adding this information to the label as a way of being different and transparent.

If the average person today starts doing some research, comparing prices and looking at transparency in labeling, they will find a huge difference in price, quality of ingredients, and the actual results as shown by testing of blood ketone levels.

We recently looked at one brand offering keto pills that contains four grams of BHB salts (Beta-hydroxybutyrate) per serving. It requires six capsules to ingest four grams of the active ingredient. There are only five servings in the entire bottle that costs $60 before tax and shipping.

Contrast this with the only exogenous ketones that we personally use and recommend, due to price, transparency in labeling, and ingredient quality and sourcing, that provides 13 grams per serving for a container of 28 servings for $50.

The consumer would spend $12 per serving to ingest four grams of BHB salts. Or they could spend less than $2 per serving to ingest 13 grams of BHB salts. The sad truth is that there are other companies offering exogenous ketones that are approaching the same cost as $12 per serving that do not even put the quantity of BHB ketone salts on the label of their products.

We would never recommend *any* of these pills for the simple reason as pointed out above on costs. We would also never recommend any exogenous ketone product that does not clearly and transparently label the quantity of ketone salts on the label.

We do believe in technology and in the advance of technology to provide new products that can improve life, results, and success transitioning into the ketogenic lifestyle. We also fully understand due diligence, testing, and finding things that work for the vast majority of people. We want to be a resource willing to seek, find and test things that improve success and offer the results and benefits that really help people.

While some people are anti-supplement, we will once again choose not to take one extreme position on either end of the spectrum. Just as we respect a person who doesn't choose to use any supplements at all, we will also remain open minded to the fact that technology advances. We will respect those who embrace technology as well. We will test new products and the results we personally get will be the determining factor on the recommendations we give.

Although we do have supplements and products that we recommend, based on personal results and benefits, we made the choice not to share them inside this book. We have a 30-Day Challenge group where we do offer our thoughts and recommendations about what supplements or other products have worked for us.

To finish this chapter, we would like to acknowledge that some people seek the ketogenic way of eating for reasons other than weight loss.

## BETSY'S STORY

Betsy Prather, systems engineer, had a diagnosis of late disseminated Lyme disease in August 1999 after having been ill for nearly 3½ years. After two treatments in an attempt at recovery, she resigned to living with illness. Then in 2001, she had her third child with which she had gestational diabetes that diet could not control. She was on insulin for the duration, placing her at an increased risk of becoming diabetic. She also lost her gallbladder just months after her child's birth.

After pregnancy and several years of living with the effects of Lyme disease, she finally found a doctor who specialized in Lyme disease who also discovered she had a Lyme co-infection. This was her first introduction to a ketogenic lifestyle. Her doctor had her begin eating ketogenic as part of his treatment because Lyme bacteria feed on sugar.

Eliminating the sugar and carbohydrates starves the bacteria. This was crucial in her healing. After 15 months on treatment, she continued to eat this way for about two more years; however, she eventually migrated back to a little more carbohydrates in her diet and then took some dietary advice from a nutritionist that had her eating carbohydrates and five to six small meals daily in an attempt to further her health goals.

After only three years of returning to eating carbohydrates and natural sugars, she received a diagnosis of early stage estrogen positive breast cancer and endured five surgeries in one year. Through much trial, error and research, she discovered that sugars and carbohydrates were responsible for increases in body fat and estrogens which had also been evident in her other health struggles with ophthalmic migraines, late onset endometriosis and borderline pre-diabetes. By removing the sugar and carbohydrates and returning to a ketogenic lifestyle, she no longer struggles with these conditions and has a heart for helping others dealing with similar health issues.

# CHAPTER 4

# The Western Diet is Killing Us

One reason the western diet is killing us is the addition of high-fructose corn syrup to foods we eat and the fact that the big food industry is adding sugar to almost anything we eat. We could write another book on how horrible this ingredient is to human beings and the effects it has had on the epidemics of obesity, diabetes and heart disease.

The quantities of sugar we are ingesting each day and each year have far surpassed what the human body is designed to process. Our blood sugar control systems are no longer able to perform as they are designed to do. Humans are consuming too much sugar at each meal, and this results in blood sugar spikes. The pancreas begins releasing insulin to get this blood sugar spike back down to normal. Insulin is the hormone that works with glucose to shuttle it into the cells of the body to create energy. When blood sugar is out of control, the excess insulin added to the system can cause the blood sugar to go lower than normal.

Low blood sugar is actually a signal to many other hormones involved with the digestive process that it is time to eat. Less than an hour after eating that meal at the Chinese restaurant, we can find our stomachs growling. We blame the Chinese food for this.

The reality is that it was the carbs ingested and the insulin spike that has driven our blood sugar from high to low that has caused these hunger pains.

We find something to snack on even while our belly is still full of undigested food. The pancreas goes into overdrive doing the job of bringing the blood sugar back down to normal. Instead of stopping perfectly at normal, the blood sugar dips low signaling that we are hungry. We have a snack. Excess calories in the body from the carb-filled foods we eat in the presence of excess insulin is the perfect condition to *store body fat*. Just think about this happening over and over again for years or decades.

Day after day we get a little fatter. Day after day we grow unhealthier. Eventually, the blood sugar control system gets so damaged that even high insulin levels will not shuttle the sugar into the cells. Our blood sugar begins to slowly increase, and even fasted blood sugar levels are high.

We get the news from our doctor that we are now type 2 diabetic and need to take medications like Metformin or Glipizide, and ultimately *more insulin* to control our blood sugar. We shrug our shoulders as we are now one more statistic who somehow "caught" type 2 diabetes. We resign ourselves to just take our medicine.

We are here to promote the simple idea that what we just described above, although the scenario has repeated itself millions of times, has failed to address the *root cause* of the problem. **Sugar.** Ingesting too much of it is the root cause. If we were not consuming the quantity of sugar that causes all the problems in the first place, our control system would work just fine. We would not have blood sugar spikes and the resulting insulin spikes that occur.

When our blood sugar dipped slightly low, it would actually be because it's time to eat some food. We would be functioning exactly as we are designed to function. It is now time for *the truth* as we understand it. *Type 2 diabetes is a choice.*

The choice we make as to what food we eat, day after day and meal after meal, is what is causing type 2 diabetes and the need for all the drugs to control blood sugar. Leaving this choice to the government, big food companies, big pharma, and the medical community is exactly what has gotten most of us into our current condition. It is time to take personal responsibility because everyone else has failed us.

Dr. Jason Fung, author of *The Diabetes Code*, puts forth the idea that type 2 diabetes is an illness of *dietary choice* being treated by medication. We have the free will to *choose* not to eat foods full of sugar. It is time that more people open up their eyes and mind to the truth.

We deeply appreciate all we have learned from Dr. Fung and his books. We pray that more of our physicians become enlightened like this amazing man. Most have focused on treating the symptoms of dietary choices with medication instead of addressing the root cause of the problem. **Sugar.** We have now experienced time and again people we personally work with minimize sugar intake and work with their doctor to reduce or eliminate medications. In fact, we expect it.

We also have the free will to keep eating what we have been eating and just take the medication. We would suggest that if you keep doing what you are doing, you will keep getting the results you have been getting. Our question to everyone we coach is: "How is that working out for you?" We believe what we are teaching is the healthier option.

Type 2 diabetes is a worldwide epidemic that will affect the health of 50% of Americans by the year 2020. Let that sink in. By 2020. That means that a family of four will have two family members with type 2 diabetes. It is just a matter of time before the number is 75%. If someone doesn't stand up and make a change, how long before the number is 100%?

Although these numbers are staggering to the point of being overwhelming, we know that the solution is extremely simple. Minimize sugar consumption.

Only **5%** of people on insulin are **type 1** insulin dependent diabetics. This means that **95%** of people using insulin are **type 2** diabetics – **95%** of people using insulin to manage the symptoms caused by *dietary choice*. There is something profoundly wrong with this. We are doing something about it.

If the food industry, big pharma, and the governments of the world had your best interest at heart this would not be the case. Why do we continue to eat this way? Why are we being taught as children that eating these foods is healthy? This blood sugar roller coaster is promoted by the food pyramid, endorsed by medical associations, and fully endorsed by big food companies and big pharma. There is no profit in wellness. The sugar roller coaster is great for the economy. It is terrible for our health and wellness.

Type 2 diabetes contributes to so many other health problems like heart disease, high blood pressure, pancreas and liver problems, diabetic ulcers, skin problems, stroke, and many more. Yet we are so addicted to sugar and carbs, we ignore the slow progression and lack of blood sugar control that occurs in our bodies as things get worse over a long period of time. This progression does not happen overnight.

Jim gets it. He had been addicted to sugar and carbs and weighed 270 pounds. Jim was not able to get his blood sugar under control no matter what he did, even with medication. Ian was on the same path with a body weight of 250 pounds at only five feet eight inches tall. We have both been stuck on the blood sugar roller coaster, not knowing that the *power of choice* was the answer for taking responsibility for our personal health.

The western diet taught us that carbs were important for energy, and breakfast is the most important meal of the day. We were told to eat smaller more frequent meals. This is all marketing designed to get you to buy and eat more food. The food is processed today so it will very strategically affect the feel-good chemicals released in your brain. There is a science of how to get people to spend more money on food, the kinds of food that keep us trapped on the blood sugar roller coaster.

It is an irrefutable fact that the system of big food companies and big pharma work hand in hand with governments to keep the economy and their balance sheets healthy. Unfortunately, your personal health is not a part or consideration in the equation. We arrived at the gut level understanding that WE are responsible for our health and wellness, not big companies and not the medical community. Certainly not the government. We decided it is up to us to be our own best healthcare advocate. Nobody else will. As long as this way of eating kills us slowly, over decades, they all get away with it.

Large chain restaurants have statistics of people who eat at their business once a month, once a week, every day, and three meals a day. This last group is referred to as "heavy users." Why do we bring this up? The fast food industry has no interest in health or quality of food you eat. These companies exist to make money. They do so with marketing and creation of foods that are designed to keep us wanting more. Nothing improves taste like deadly sugar.

The cravings and experience keep us coming back for more over and over again. Add the fact that we can pull into a drive-through window on just about any block in town and have an order ready in minutes and we have developed the recipe for the diabetes and obesity epidemic.

Every day we are being bombarded with advertisements for snacks, fast food, and sugary sodas. This is one of the reasons we have a growing obesity epidemic. When everything you eat has no nutritional value and contains massive quantities of sugar, there is a problem. We have been the guinea pigs for an amazing advertising and marketing plan that is making lots of profit for these companies at the cost of the health of the vast majority of people.

One of the major reasons the current obesity/diabetes/heart disease epidemic started is that George McGovern signed a bill in 1974 called the Government Dietary Guidelines sponsored and lobbied for by the food industry. This formed the food pyramid for our public schools. So as children we were taught to eat plenty of carbohydrates. That's right, kids. *You need to eat more sugar!*

Sugar addiction was guaranteed and sanctioned by the government to start at a very early age. The ADA and American Heart Association support these guidelines. Do you think there's an agenda? This is the system we deal with.

The pattern we see looking back at history is that government told us what to eat, and it is clear to see by any reasonable person that eating that way causes humans to get sicker over time; but not to worry as the drug companies are pumping the drugs out to keep your symptoms medicated. We humans may not be healthy, but the economy certainly is.

Medical science has proven that if you quit ingesting carbs and sugar, your pancreas and liver will repair itself. Simply correcting *what* we eat will correct the obesity and diabetes epidemics. A few simple changes can literally change your life and health. Please take in the following information and really let it sink in. The quantities of sugar that the average person ingests is *staggering.* This is the root cause of the problem of diabetes and obesity.

The Western European sugar industry was born in the mid-1600s, and in a very short period of human history has now grown to be the third most valuable crop after cereals and rice. Back in the 1600s, sugar was only available to the wealthy elite. Sugar was a very small part of the human diet with only seasonal pulses from fruits and vegetables locally grown or foraged.

By 1700, average consumption of sugar in the developed world increased to approximately *four pounds of sugar* per year, accounting for less than *1%* of calorie intake. By 1800, this number increased to approximately *18 pounds* per year and by 1900, it was *60 pounds* per year. Currently, just 119 years later, according to the American government, the average American ingests *152 pounds of sugar per year.* This is a staggering number. *Nearly three pounds per week.*

Although the human body is amazingly adaptive, the truth is that our built-in blood sugar control system is not designed to process this sickening amount of sugar. One of the main reasons for this proliferation of sugar consumption was the invention of soda. In the late 1800s to early 1900s, the mass production of all our favorite sodas began. Where sugar had been afforded only by the elite until then, mass production brought cheap soda filled with sugar to the masses. *One can* of soda contains about *11 teaspoons of sugar.*

We don't believe any reasonable person would dump 11 teaspoons of sugar into a glass of water or tea and drink it down, yet many people don't have a second thought about drinking multiple full-sugar sodas every day. This shows how easy it is to have no idea how much sugar we consume, and this is just one product. This sad reality is taking a toll on our health that seems to get worse every year, and people stay oblivious.

This is affecting every area of our life, especially the cost of healthcare. Today we have children with type 2 diabetes. *Children!* This is a scary statistic. We have new parents shoving bottles of pure sugar fruit juice or soda into their child's mouth, having zero understanding of the health consequences that child will be paying later. They are growing them into our next crop of type 2 diabetics. We are sure that the big food, big pharma, and those who make a living treating the symptoms appreciate this early training. It seems that if we keep creating more type 2 diabetics, they will keep selling the drugs to medicate the symptoms of our dietary choices.

It is difficult enough to make the right choices and overcome this early childhood training that carbs are *good*, but it can be even more difficult when we believe we are making a better choice, only to be confused by ingredients on the label, especially when deemed "healthy" by organizations supposedly looking out for the public.

Jim decided to have a keto snack and chose a bag of pork rinds. It was super low in carbs, according to the label. After having his snack, Jim checked his blood sugar and found it had spiked to 250! The brand he chose contained *maltodextrin*. The point of this discussion is to get everyone to understand that you must become your own advocate and learn about these ingredients. Spend a minute to read a label. Keep a list in your phone of all the names the government allows these companies to use instead of the word sugar. These are the new habits we must form as we take the First Steps 2 Keto.

## Corn and high-fructose corn syrup

We could write an entire book about this horrible ingredient and the health effects it is having on human beings. Suffice to say, with a little research we believe any reasonable person would come to the same conclusion. High-fructose corn syrup is horrible for human beings. Anyone who suggests otherwise is in complete denial.

One of the largest crops in America is corn and it is used to make high-fructose corn syrup, an inexpensive sweetener used in many packaged foods. The problem with high-fructose corn syrup is it is absorbed like sugar but metabolizes like alcohol increasing fatty liver by 37%. We believe that this sugar substitute that is added to so many foods is causing type 2 diabetes at an accelerated rate. As long as we continue to eat processed and packaged food, our health will continue to decline. Awareness of how unhealthy this ingredient is and making the choice not to put it in our bodies is an option for better health.

It is no wonder that our kids are getting type 2 diabetes. This was unheard of until after 1970, and that's not that long ago. In less than 40 years, we have created a generation of young people who are dealing with a preventable disease caused entirely by diet. This is madness on every level. Here is where we have a problem with what we call the "sugar agenda."

We do not believe it is by chance that food now has more sugar for taste than at any other time in history when the number one ingredient in processed food is high-fructose corn syrup or when maltodextrin is an additive in products that should not have sugar, like pork rinds. This is all for taste and compels people to crave the food and eat more. Many of these ingredients are also designed and created to bypass the feedback loop that tells the brain we are full, and it is time to stop eating. This is insanity, but it is 100% true.

When food tastes good and releases those feel-good chemicals in the brain, you will crave more. Sugar releases dopamine, a neurotransmitter involved in reward-based behavior. Studies are showing that sugar is more addictive than cocaine. This is good news for the food industry. This is how every year they sell more food. The prices keep going up, and we keep paying. See where we are going with this, friends?

At some point we must become our own best advocates. It is our responsibility. The sugar agenda is real. Not only is big food benefiting from sugar addiction, but it goes hand in hand with big pharma. Insulin is a $42 billion a year industry and growing every year. This all stems from one thing: the change in sugar consumption in the western diet. This is why we are rotting from the inside out.

You may say, "Well, Ian and Jim, that's all great to know but how do I get off this sugar roller coaster, this never-ending cycle, and this dietary choice that has been leading to sick care instead of healthcare?"

It's not easy, friend, but it is fairly simple. There is *hope*. It is called First Steps 2 Keto.

## CHRISTINA'S STORY

Christina Chaney-Smith was introduced to Ian through a mutual friend in early 2016. He attempted to share some information about getting started with the ketogenic lifestyle, and Christina immediately decided Ian was just trying to sell her stuff. She just wasn't ready.

During this time, Christina got married, and even as her weight continued to increase, she was blessed with the news they were expecting. What should have been a joyous time was full of anxiety as she wondered if her weight would be bad for the baby. Christina and her husband were blessed with a healthy baby boy in 2017, yet post-partum depression affected her. Now at the heaviest weight of her life, Christina was embarrassed to even leave the house and would only do so for appointments for her son. Christina cried every time she saw her reflection in the mirror.

Christina prayed a prayer. Not for herself, but a prayer to be a blessing to others. If God would help her lose weight and become healthier, her prayer was that it would be to the benefit of others. Within three days of her prayer, the information she needed to hear started coming from multiple directions. Ask and ye shall receive. Christina reconnected with Ian and joined their keto support group. Christina stayed open minded and did anything she could to learn and help other new members.

She shared her experiences and her challenges with the hope of getting a new person more success. She became open to testing out new products such as electrolytes and smart chocolate. She began to identify what did and did not work for her. Ian asked Christina to help him and Betsy by becoming an admin of the keto group and she accepted, and is now considered family.

It might also be important to mention that over this time Christina released over 113 pounds from her body. She is now a totally different person, and her prayer continues to be answered as she works tirelessly to support the newest person just getting started.

# CHAPTER 5

# We Are Designed to Eat Ketogenic

Humans are designed to eat ketogenic. Our ancestors have been hunter gatherers since the dawn of time. As far back in time as cavemen roamed the earth, we have hunted, fished and foraged for edible natural foods.

What we have witnessed over and over again as we have worked with others to transition to the ketogenic lifestyle is the fact that when humans start eating the way our bodies were designed, the way our hunter/gatherer ancestors did, the body starts to heal itself.

Ancient tribes, Inuit Indians, and tribes of the rain forest did not deal with these modern medical issues until they started eating the western diet full of sugar and processed crap. The aboriginal people of Australia are well documented as being lean and healthy. When they started eating the western diet, and all the sugar involved, they started experiencing the same health issues of heart disease, diabetes and obesity. Check out the documentary *The Magic Pill* to see this for yourself. As this population begins to eat the foods of their ancestors, healing and health return.

# The Inuit paradox

The indigenous tribes and inhabitants of the northernmost villages thrived on mostly fat and protein from animals hunted or fished for. This was the way of life for thousands of years until modern man started relocating and building towns and cities that brought the Industrial Revolution to these remote areas.

Inupiat and Yupiks of Alaska, the Canadian Inuit and Inuvialuit, Inuit Greenlanders and Siberian Yupiks rarely had the opportunity to forage for roots. The occasional treat of berries during the subarctic summer was indeed a rare treat. There was no dairy. There were no vegetable gardens or 24-hour grocery stores to buy these items. How did this population survive over all that time without the "balanced diet" the governments, big food companies, and every diet guru out there seem to insist upon?

Why is it that when these people started to partake in this amazing "balanced" diet they started suffering the same ill effects as the rest of humanity: heart disease, type 2 diabetes and obesity. We can write for hours about all of the research studying this topic, but we recommend you do some for yourself. All of the evidence is readily available and plain to see if anyone cares to actually take a look. This is when becoming your own best advocate and doing your own research can be immensely powerful. *Google is your friend.* Do some research!

One of the most important take-aways from researching the diets of indigenous tribes is the reality that eating only meat, especially lean protein, was not healthy for these indigenous people either. Healthy fat is what they ate. These indigenous people had diets of greater than 50% of calories from animal fat and fat from cold-water fish and other creatures from the sea.

Let's face facts. Since the 1950s, dietary fat has been demonized. We have been told that fat plugs up arteries and causes heart attacks.

Eating fat makes you fat. Fat is the cause of all of the health issues we face. The government, the medical establishment, big pharma all jumped on the low-fat, high-carbohydrate diet bandwagon.

We now have epidemic levels of obesity, heart disease and diabetes. We have younger people being diagnosed with these issues every single year that goes by. And the other important statistic that just keeps increasing? *Sugar consumption.* It is like the big giant elephant in the room that is conveniently ignored. We are told we should just exercise more and take our medication.

# Industrial Revolution

## Moving off the farm and into the cities

Another easily researched part of history is the Industrial Revolution. Starting in the late 1700s in Britain, and then moving around the world in the 1800s and into the 1900s, this 200-year time frame of world history completely changed society around the world. Like all things human, some things improved and some things suffered. To cover this time in simplistic terms for the purpose of this book, we want to discuss a couple of facts.

At the time the Industrial Revolution began, most people lived in rural areas, around small townships, and grew their own crops, hunted and fished for meat, and raised animals for their own food supply. Manufacturing of any sort was done at home with hand tools. The Industrial Revolution saw an explosion of technology as textiles expanded, followed by metallurgy improvements in cast iron production that gave way to mass produced steel. Iron and steel became essential materials that led to mass production of tools and machines that enabled mass production of appliances, machines, ships, and larger buildings and other infrastructure.

The Revolution continued into transportation as steam engines, including trains and steamboats, began altering shipping and transportation of goods across the world. Followed soon by mass production of the automobile, business of all kinds started booming and more and more factories were being built in every imaginable industry. These factories and employers needed employees.

Factories were built near larger cities because this is where the transportation hubs were located. More people started migrating away from the small family farms and relocating in urban areas. As fewer people were growing crops, big companies started following the rest of the business community and started mass-producing the food supply. Just as the small family farm profited from a good harvest, the big food companies were born and focused on the same goal.

A company's existence is about making a profit. Like many other issues arising from the Industrial Revolution, there are many amazing benefits and technological advances that came to the food industry. At the same time, there were many negative growing pains learned in all industries.

For the purposes of this book, we will point out that there is so much history to learn from if you take the time to do a little research. The simple version here is that the Industrial Revolution resulted in a mass migration of humans around the earth, including America, still in infancy as a country, whereby people moved from small rural family farms to bigger cities where the factories were being built and companies needed employees. Because of this, many people that used to work their own land as families became less active, and they turned over the quality of their food to other people, including big companies that have only grown bigger over time and had increasing control over the quality of food on the market and the ingredients in the food.

The golden rule is the truth here. He who has the gold makes the rules. Big money lobbies governments. Large donations can sway teaching at institutions of higher learning. Money can influence research, what is clinically studied, what the results of studies are and who they favor.

Many alignments happened that caused the government to put out the food pyramid, for the ever-increasing carbohydrate count to begin its steady upward trend, and for dietary fat to start being demonized as the cause of all health problems.

## Big business, academia and government start manipulating the public

As reported in major news organizations in summer of 2016, internal sugar industry documents discovered by a university researcher at the University of California, San Francisco and published in JAMA Internal Medicine, exposed five decades of research concerning nutrition and heart disease that was manipulated by the sugar industry. "How in the world could that happen?" you may ask.

The documents exposed a trade group called the Sugar Research Foundation, currently called the Sugar Association, who paid cash money to Harvard Scientist to publish papers on fat, sugar, and their role in heart disease. The studies used were targeted by the sugar trade group to demonize fat and be lenient on sugar. The results were published in the *New England Journal of Medicine*.

The scientists from Harvard have all since passed away but it is interesting to note that one of them, Dr. Mark Hegsted, went on to be appointed as the Head of Nutrition at the U.S. Department of Agriculture. In 1977, he just so happened to help draft what became the federal government's dietary guidelines. In our opinion, these guidelines put out by the government can be pointed to as one of the absolute main reasons for the explosion of obesity, diabetes and heart disease that continues all these decades later.

Another of the scientists was Dr. Fredrick J. Stare, Chairman of Harvard's nutrition department. Apparently, the review was published at a time when medical journals did not require researchers to disclose who was funding the research. It was not until the mid-1980s that the *New England Journal of Medicine* started to require such disclosures.

The Sugar Association still contends that despite this lack of funding transparency for several decades, their research has concluded that sugar "does not have a unique role in heart disease."

Add to this many other historical documents that showed big companies in the soda and candy industry downplayed the role of sugary sodas in the role of obesity and that children that ate candy actually weighed less than children who didn't.

Isn't that amazing? Candy (sugar) is so healthy it would actually cause children to lose weight. Documents from the 1960s show top sugar executives discussed with others in the sugar industry a plan to shift and shape public opinion "through our research, information and legislative programs."

If you continue to disbelieve the reality that these big companies have manipulated everything, from those in the government (legislative), the education system itself (information, bogus studies, etc. including false research) and the medical establishment, it's time to wake up to the truth. They did it for one reason. **Profit.** The fact that studies and research were skewed in this way was a direct result of the golden rule. Once again, those with all the gold made up their own rules as they went along.

At the same time this sugar whitewash was happening, the anti-fat lobby was just taking off. Ancel Keys may be the single human who had the most influence over this conversation at the time. The Minnesota physiologist put forth his theory that saturated fat and dietary cholesterol were the culprits of heart disease and he set out to prove his theory true, beginning in the late 1950s.

There is an ongoing heated debate about Ancel Keys' Seven Countries Study which concluded with his finding that saturated fat in the diet causes plugged arteries, heart disease and heart attacks. In simple terms, the countries in his study that ate the highest amount of fat also had the most heart disease. It has been pointed out by those who disagree with his findings that many countries that consume high amounts of fat, but *do not* have more heart disease, were conveniently omitted. The argument is that he wanted to find a certain conclusion, and he only allowed data into the study that would prove his theory.

Those who agree with him and his findings vehemently defend his methods and data with excuses why these other countries were omitted, and when some of the groups that support his findings are investigated, it has been shown that many of them have their own agenda such as promoting veganism, etc.

We have stated in the book that we are just a couple of regular guys. We are not highly educated men. We are highly experienced at eating the Standard American Diet and suffering the physical health results of it. We have done our best to be our own best advocates. We have done our best to use the resources available to do our own research into this and many other issues we believe are affecting our fellow human's health.

Sometimes it can be very difficult as these different sides and extremes make their arguments for and against these controversial studies and findings, especially when highly educated academics, doctors and other really smart people weigh in and nobody seems to agree. It depends on what you stand for, and the stakes in this argument are simply huge.

We will give our opinion that the mission of the sugar industry has been, since the 1950s, to just keep things inconclusive. As long as the finger wasn't pointed at them, that was good enough. The results affect big food companies, big pharma, and the medical establishment. For decades the sugar industry has done anything it can to distort and deflect the role of sugar in having any negative effects on obesity, heart disease or diabetes. This is an undisputed fact, based on the documents discovered that we wrote about previously.

And since Ancel Keys' death in 2004, the distortions and deflections continue to muddy up the waters about who is to blame for the epidemic of obesity, heart disease and diabetes we have witnessed around the world, and there is no dispute that these epidemics are happening.

We are a couple of simple guys, who ate what they told us to eat, as is taught on the food pyramid, that has been taught in school to children for decades. We both got horribly fat and sick, just like the growing majority of humans that are eating the Standard American Diet. We try to keep things simple for the sake of understanding.

Here is a question for you. What do you get when you mix flour, sugar and oil (fat)?

Cake batter!! We believe and have witnessed that mixing these ingredients in the human body creates its own special cake batter in the arteries. Yes, we agree 100% that eating a diet that combines all these ingredients together is the recipe for obesity, heart disease and diabetes.

Regardless of what countries Ancel Keys did or didn't pick for his study, and regardless of whether he actually cherry-picked the seven he chose so that it would guarantee the results he wanted, we want to point out what he apparently **did not** take into account in his study. That is the undisputed fact that from the late 1800s, when sugar started being delivered very cheaply to the masses in the form of soda, until the late 1950s when Keys started his study, all the way until his death in 2004, concluding with the modern day you are reading this book, the daily consumption of sugar has continued to increase.

This consumption has continued to increase in every country that Keys included in his study as well as those he excluded. We very simply believe that it is the combinations of sugar and fat that have caused the health epidemics we are witnessing.

We base this belief on the undeniable fact that we have now experienced so many times, with so many different people, that when these humans make the choice to eliminate or minimize consumption of sugar, better health is the result. We can say with certainty the result of eliminating fat is not the same. The high-carb, low-fat diet recommended for decades is a large part of our obesity, heart disease and diabetes epidemics.

When people stop ingesting sugar, there are some amazing health benefits that occur. The blood sugar roller coaster *stops* happening. Blood sugar levels calm down and stop swinging up and down. When blood sugar calms down, the resulting insulin spikes also calm down. These people stop repeatedly putting themselves into fat storage mode. If their blood sugar dips a little low, it is because it is actually time to eat.

We have witnessed these humans release all the extra water weight they are carrying around caused by the consumption of sugar. Releasing this extra fluid in the form of water weight is beneficial for a number of health issues. For every gram of carb consumed, the body can hold on to four grams of water. This is an indicator that sustaining a low-carb lifestyle is important to keep this water weight off.

When sugar is restricted at low enough levels for a long enough period of time, the body will begin releasing stored body fat into the bloodstream, processing the fat in the liver, and creating ketone bodies. These chemical molecules are able to enter at the cellular level and create energy, just like glucose does.

This ketogenesis, or the creation of ketones from fat, is the mechanism that causes fat loss in the ketogenic lifestyle. Reducing body fat and weight to healthy levels provides so many benefits to overall health. Ketones are actually proven to create almost 40% more energy per unit of oxygen at the cellular level. Ketones are proven to have amazing anti-inflammatory properties. Ketones are amazingly neuro-protective, and elevating blood ketone levels by restricting carbs was the preferred method to treat epilepsy in children and adults starting in the 1920s causing a reduction or even elimination of seizures in children and adults.

Adding up the positive results of minimizing sugar from the diet looks like this:

*Calms down and normalizes blood sugar swings and insulin response to those swings.

*Releases excess water weight.

*Begins ketogenesis, utilizing fat for fuel and body weight comes down.

*Blood sugar numbers normalize and improve.

*As blood ketone levels increase, many people experience improved energy levels and cognitive benefits, as well as the neuro-protective properties of ketones.

*As body weight comes down to healthier levels, blood sugar normalizes and energy levels improve, people tend to feel better and become more active.

*As people get down to maintenance weight, and the body stops releasing as much stored fat into the blood, we see people who had horrible cholesterol numbers improving and normalization of blood lipid numbers, most importantly particle size of LDL cholesterol becomes larger and "fluffy" and does not stick together causing plugs.

The smaller sticky particles are no longer present, and most importantly the inflammation all throughout the body that more and more enlightened doctors are recognizing as the main cause of all disease and illness, including in the arterial walls, is reduced or eliminated.

We have seen personal blood work, and had many other people share their blood work results that have had huge improvements in liver enzymes and fatty liver issues by simply reducing or minimizing sugar in the diet. Even after being warned that eating healthy fat would worsen fatty liver, the exact opposite occurred when sugar was removed. We have seen it with our own eyes time and time again that when inflammatory sugar is removed or minimized, the body begins healing itself. Inflammation subsides, and all health markers of inflammation improve.

We have also witnessed time and again that people decide to get started in the ketogenic lifestyle, and they do so with no baseline blood work. They have no idea where they started. Then for some reason or another, they go to their doctor and inform them that they are eating ketogenic. Despite any progress made to that point, the doctors often times want to do blood work and check cholesterol, liver enzymes, etc.

Also, despite the fact that often times it is decades of eating the Standard American Diet that has brought the person to their current level of health crisis, whatever negative results that come back with the blood work are blamed on the new ketogenic way of eating.

We believe it is dishonest, shortsighted and lazy on the part of anyone who would blame decades of poor food choices results on a short-term change in eating. We also believe that when these people have been stable at maintenance weight for three months, blood work will actually show the "new normal." The body is no longer releasing extra stored body fat into the blood. Blood lipid readings normalize.

If you are the kind of person who is going to be intimidated by treatment such as this, we strongly encourage you to be your own best advocate for personal health and wellness. You must develop the mindset that until you are at maintenance level for three months, the current readings are *temporary*.

We suggest getting this blood work done from the beginning to establish a baseline or starting point of reclaiming your personal health. We also suggest taking an honest look at what your heathy goal weight should be, and because we suggest not setting a weight loss goal for more than one pound per week, it should be simple math to calculate how many weeks it should take to achieve this goal. We personally would not worry or stress about blood work results until that weight loss goal is met, personal macros are met, and maintenance calories are dialed in to maintain that goal weight. We have been a witness to all numbers totally normalizing within a few months of dialing all this in.

Here is the truth. If you didn't pay attention to how horrible your numbers were on blood work until this point, why should you do so now? Especially knowing this is a short-term situation to get your health back and on track.

If you do have a baseline and see the numbers get worse after starting ketogenic eating, it is realistic to understand that utilizing body fat for fuel is going to release it into the bloodstream where it can be converted into ketones. It would only stand to reason that blood lipids would increase during this time.

Once at maintenance, the body will not have all this fat to release into the bloodstream. It stands to reason these blood lipids would decrease. We are advocating to give yourself a chance in the short term. Look at the facts. Doing what you have done has gotten you your current results. Be honest about the amount of time it has taken you to get to this point. If a person has 50 pounds to lose, they know it's going to take approximately 50 weeks.

Settle in and realize that 50 weeks to get to maintenance weight is short term compared to the decades of Standard American Diet that got you to this point. Take responsibility for your personal health and wellness. Arm yourself with this mindset.

There are those people in various fields who adamantly refuse to accept the results and benefits of the ketogenic way of eating. It is our mission to continue to share the truth, one person at a time, through every means at our disposal, to do our best to educate these people and provide them with better information. We want to understand their motivation for refusing to accept that ketogenic eating is the way we were designed to live.

Sugar is not inherently evil, yet we hope we have shown in this chapter that man is capable of manipulation, in the interest of profit, to create the truth you need to see to be a good consumer and make him lots of profit, even at the expense of your long-term health.

Higher education is capable of manipulation with money. Scientific studies are manipulated to produce the results that benefit those paying for the study. The public isn't funding these studies, big companies do. Big pharma is right there to create another drug that everyone needs to take.

The medical field is simply doing what they are taught. If you question your personal doctor about the actual hours spent studying nutrition in college, don't be shocked when it amounts to a couple of hours of their time. Add to that the fact that big business is behind the funding of this education, and these doctors are simply practicing what they were taught.

When the medical field is rewarded for writing those prescriptions and it becomes a part of their financial compensation, as well as a source of funding for the education they received, it isn't that difficult to acknowledge that we have a system in place that works hand in hand at the various levels from big business, the medical establishment, the educational system, and the governments of the world to profit from the system at the expense of the public health.

We believe it is time to put the actual health and wellness of people ahead of these profits. We are not anti-business, or anti-doctor, or even anti-government. We are against the system that has been profiting off the sugar agenda for decades. Perhaps this warrants a large-scale study, conducted by an unbiased third party, which demonstrates what actually happens to people when they minimize sugar in the diet.

What happens to the dosages of medications they are taking to control blood sugar and blood pressure? What happens to cholesterol numbers when these people reach their maintenance weight and keep it there? We doubt it would happen because we are already seeing the results.

## ANTHONY'S STORY

Anthony Galetto is your New York City, Italian, single dad American who joined the Navy and served his country. That's where he met Jim. 9/11, 2001 changed everything. Anthony was out of the Navy but ended up spending months as a first responder at Ground Zero. Anthony re-enlisted and served again through Operation Iraqi Freedom.

After leaving the Navy for the second time, Anthony was employed as an engineer for a prominent hotel in Times Square. Since 2012 he suffered three different injuries, all requiring surgery. Out of 84 months, 33 of them were spent recovering from surgery; 33 months is a lot of time staring at the walls, thinking too much, getting depressed. Anthony had nothing to do but think and eat, and both were feeding his PTSD.

In June of 2018, his old Navy buddy Jim reached out to Anthony to share with him what ketogenic eating had done for him. Vets look out for each other, as it's a known fact that they have lost a lot of brothers to PTSD. Jim shared some things he had found that were really working for him.

At this time, Anthony was sitting at home, pending approval for torn ACL and MCL. Workers Comp was taking their time and Anthony was in a lot of pain. Anthony told Jim straight up, "I don't have time to entertain gimmicks."

By January 2019, with little improvement in the knee after surgery and feeling defeated, Anthony was almost 190 pounds at five feet three inches tall. The symptoms of PTSD he had always been able to bury or ignore started escalating into anxiety and panic attacks that Anthony had never experienced before.

Fortunately, Jim noticed these changes and in a way only brothers at arms can do, informed Anthony that he was about to go keto and learn about Smart Coffee. Anthony agreed, and within two short weeks his entire life, mental state, outlook and mindset did a complete 180-degree turn. Anthony felt *awakened*.

Restoration came not only mentally but also physically as he minimized the sugar intake. Anthony was down 30 pounds in less than four months, and he now feels better mentally and physically than he did in his 20s.

Anthony joined Jim and Ian in the original First Steps 2 Keto 30-Day Challenge and quickly realized that he loves sharing what he has learned with others in the group. It still seems amazing just how fast things have turned around.

Realizing how many other people are out there suffering in silence, Anthony decided to start working with other new people and teach what he has learned. Sometimes it is very difficult to understand why good people go through such difficult things until that experience is able to help another person in a way nothing else could.

# CHAPTER 6

# Don't Compare Your Journey to Anyone Else

Comparison is the thief of joy. We are all different. You will hear us repeat this mantra over and over again. We are all different.

One of the biggest downfalls we see is when people start comparing their results to other people. We are all different. Different genders, ages, stress levels, activity levels, food consumption, level of seriousness, different motivations, different reasons *why* we are seeking the results and benefits of the ketogenic lifestyle, different hormone issues, and different metabolisms.

What may be the absolute best choice for one person may be the very thing that does not work at all for another. One person may cut carbs back to 50 grams a day and get great results, while another person cuts carbs back to 20 grams per day and doesn't seem to be making any progress. One person seems to get unrealistic crazy results because they drop a bunch of water weight initially while another person struggles to lose any weight at all. Why is this? It is because we are all different.

We have also witnessed many people who are obese that really don't eat much food. They do not fit the stereotypical idea of an overweight person who are just gluttons who eat too much food at every meal. When we dig deeper, we discover that many of these people simply cut back more thinking it was going to help with weight loss.

Instead, to combat their weight, they cut back on portion sizes, some cut back numbers of meals, and some people cut back to eating one small meal a day. These people have trained their metabolism to slow down to the point their body is holding on to any calories that it takes in.

These people have no energy level or motivation to get up and move. They don't feel good. Sometimes these patterns have been practiced for years, and many times it has been practiced for decades. These metabolic issues are not like light switches that get flipped on or off. These are patterns that have become homeostasis. Their "normal" has got to be retrained and put into a higher gear. The good news is that the human body is amazing at being able to reset.

Everyone is different, and we would caution those who get fast results and want to brag about those results to anyone who will listen that you are now "doing keto" and losing weight fast and that keto is the easiest thing you have ever done. As fast as you got results, you can also get negative results just as fast. We have heard it thousands of times. It is people just like these that seem to disappear the fastest. Stopping doing the easiest thing they ever did puts that weight right back on just as fast as it came off. Generally speaking, these fast results are water weight that naturally comes off due to restricting carb intake. This water will be retained just as it was before if this person ingests sugar again.

Everyone is different, and what is really more important than fast results is knowing that our bodies are designed for the ketogenic lifestyle, and we call it a *lifestyle instead of a diet*. Eating this way really is a way of life because when we stop doing it, we get exactly the same results we had before. We get inflammation, water retention (which is a really fast way to gain weight) and fat storage, instead of using fat for fuel. Most people feel like garbage, the authors included, when we make the choice to consume sugar. Some of us have made those choices anyway. We are human, too. We are not perfect and we have suffered the consequences of these poor choices.

We believe choices like this are made due to "euphoric recall." In the same way, drug addicts and alcoholics relapse because their brains can only seem to recall the good times and the fun times but seem incapable of recalling how horrible things really got. This is something we all go through during our journey, and we suggest that it's not *if* it happens, but *when.*

The most important thing will be how you react and respond. Do you get back with your program of better health and wellness? Or are you the kind of person that allows a bite of cake to turn into a cheat meal that evolves into a cheat day, cheat week, or cheat month? *Know thyself.* It is so important to be honest with yourself. If you know this is how you respond, it would be important to focus on that rather than some euphoric recall memories from days gone by.

## Your macros are the only macros that matter

Because everyone is different, there is no need to compare your personal macros to anyone else. These macro numbers are based on some complicated calculations that take age, gender, height, activity level, current weight and body type into consideration. Please remember that as your weight comes down, your macros will have to be reset every 15-20 pounds lost. Your current weight has changed and so will your personal macros.

Some people may get to eat more calories. Some may eat less. There will be differing amounts of grams of fats, protein and carbs. None of this information matters at all. The only thing that matters is *your* macros, unless you are helping someone else in your household because you are preparing meals and their macros are different.

Take the focus off of anyone else and put it in the most important place. That place to focus is on yourself. Get yourself comfortable using the calculator and apps to know your personal macros and reset them when needed to stay on track and not stall out. As your weight comes down, your calorie requirements to support that weight also come down. Continuing to eat a caloric amount based on a heavier weight will cause you to stall and stop losing weight.

One side effect we have seen with some who start eating ketogenic is a loss of appetite. While this may seem preferable to previous experience with other diets where we stayed hungry all the time, the fact is that we must take in enough calories or we risk shunting the metabolism. The body doesn't know the difference between starvation on purpose or by choice. The body understands survival. It will hang on to any calories taken in and store as long as possible in this starvation mode.

We suggest knowing your personal macros, and eating the required caloric intake based on your goal. If you do not take in enough calories you risk stalling out your weight loss. This is totally defeating the purpose of those eating ketogenic to burn off excess body fat. This is important information to know as it affects our mindset. Our minds can distract us and taking the focus off ourselves and putting the focus on other people is one way this distraction can happen. We have to work on **our** mindset.

## Mindset

We have found that developing a positive mindset is key. This life can be tough and we all go through challenges on a daily basis. Making positive mindset a priority, simply by taking a few minutes a day to meditate, pray, listen to some positive motivational speakers, reading a chapter of a positive personal development book, and most importantly writing a gratitude list, makes such a profound impact on us and others that we have to mention it in this book.

There is so much negativity in the world, and with the 24-hour news cycles, print media and access to the internet on our phones, we are all inundated with thousands of negative images and stories every single day. It is easy to be totally consumed and affected by all of this negativity. For those of us who stress eat, or eat to just feel better, staying consumed and wrapped up in negative energy and influence is not healthy for us.

Ian and his wife Betsy had many things in common when they met. Both of them had stopped watching television years before meeting. Other than an occasional movie or documentary (like *The Magic Pill* – please watch this documentary if you have not seen it) we simply avoid the television, the news, and focus on more positive things in life that we do have control over.

We make the choice to read good books or listen to the audio version. We take the time to go for walks or go to the gym and work out together because it is a positive self-loving service to our bodies. We choose to go to church and fill our hearts and souls up with positive input.

We do continuous acts of service, the kinds of things you just don't hear about on the news. We give to causes we believe in, like our friend who rescues baby animals and cares for them until they can be released. This makes our hearts happy. We support an orphanage and educational system in a foreign country that our church supports. We support our amazing friend who has been a missionary in India for almost a decade, because our hearts call us to support the amazing things this woman has accomplished half a world away.

Why do we include this in a book about the ketogenic lifestyle? We do so because mindset matters! Releasing the negativity and making room for the positive matters!

Ultimately, what has transpired in the lives of both Ian and Jim is that we first worked on getting our personal health in order. We then made the decision to start sharing what we had learned to the best of our ability. We have found that working to improve the health and wellness of other people has become one of the greatest sources of helping ourselves.

It has not been easy, or painless, and we have had to thicken our own skin. We deal with decades of disinformation that has been taught to us all. We deal with the attitudes and beliefs of the gym world. This is something else entirely.

Despite all of the possible negativity we face, other people's opinions and belief systems, what we discovered was that this exchange of information and building of community has been the greatest source of healing ourselves. It has taught us both the ultimate truth of giving to receive. We strongly suggest that as you take the simple First Steps 2 Keto and get started, focus on healing yourself, but share what you are experiencing with others who are going through the same experience.

Being involved in a group of people doing the same thing at the same time as you can be the perfect opportunity to share challenges, ask questions, give and receive encouragement. There is power in building a community like this.

## Finding what works for YOU!

Developing a positive mindset is also really important for dealing with any personal challenges that you may face. It could be hormone issues, or it could be dealing with family or spouse that is not supportive, or a work environment where people don't want to see you succeed.

We call this last one the "crabs in a bucket" environment. Sometimes the people around you don't mind seeing you do well, they just mind when they see you do better than them. When a person makes the choice to take responsibility for improving their health and actually starts producing positive results, the people around them can start sabotaging and become negative and unsupportive. Just like the crab trying to escape the bucket of poor health, the other crabs start pulling you back down with them.

It seems that we all have to go through obstacles and challenges like this of one kind or another. It is almost like a rite of passage we all have to go through to determine how badly we really want better health and wellness. We can use it to grow stronger in our beliefs, or we can allow this negative energy to pull us back down in the bucket.

We sincerely hope you choose to grow stronger and rise above the negativity. How you respond to your personal challenges is what is really important. If you don't have to deal with challenges like this from those close to you in your life, that is okay too. We mention this because we have seen this type of negative response. We have seen this response from people we did not expect it from. We have also seen it from those in the medical profession as well as the news media, sometimes from utterly bizarre sources, and even from a person's spouse or family or best friend.

When it does happen, from whatever source, we have to learn to thicken our skin. It helps to seek to understand rather than demand to be understood. At the same time, we are having to focus on the foundation of our belief in what we are doing and the changes we are making.

We have to have a strong enough belief in the ketogenic lifestyle to withstand any negative that may be directed at us. We suggest you base it off results instead of opinions or what the latest news report, magazine article, or celebrity trainer has to say. You have to understand the motives behind the negativity.

We have found that many times you can just follow the money. Or in some cases we have seen people seeking attention for themselves by being a negative voice or opinion against something so obviously benefitting the vast majority of people who honestly put the ketogenic lifestyle to the test. Choose carefully who you get your information from and begin building a strong foundation to your lifestyle. We hope and pray that we give you good information through First Steps 2 Keto.

## Help yourself to be a blessing to others

Taking personal responsibility for your health can be a very solitary idea at first, especially for some of us who have tried and failed too many times at every conceivable "diet." We count ourselves amongst those who felt we had tried everything and failed.

Having failed at everything before, we find it easy to expect to fail again. This history does not inspire confidence for us to share our choices with the world. They have all been a witness to our many failures as well. We totally relate to this mindset. We have trained our thinking and expectations in advance based on past experience. We believe each of us that begins a very personal journey with a unique story can make the choice to focus on ourselves and take responsibility for our personal health. This foundation is important. Learning and putting the correct information into personal practice is key to building a strong foundation for the ketogenic lifestyle.

We also ask you to be open to sharing your story, what you have learned that is working, and the results and benefits you have found by implementing what you have learned. Our hope and prayer are that you find out, as we did, that being open to give what you have learned will bless you as you receive the powerful gift of witnessing other people regain their personal health and wellness. There will always be a fine line between being a know-it-all and sharing information with someone who is asking for it.

# CHAPTER 7

# Ketogenic Eating is Not a Cost, It's an Investment

Being members of the keto community for years now, building online communities on social media and experimenting with different ways to teach, share, and deliver content to people wanting to learn the ketogenic lifestyle, one of the recurring themes we hear over and over is, "Why is keto so expensive?"

We have taken a deep look at this topic. We took an inward look at our own experience as well as an outward look at the changes that have occurred in supplement or support product technology, the options now available for ketogenic foods or ingredients available, as well as options available while on the road or eating at restaurants.

Paying for quality is always going to be more expensive. We are going to suggest that *dollar menu mentality* is exactly what got most of us in the health condition that we were in before the ketogenic lifestyle. We propose that it is time to elevate our thinking and mindset about what our health is worth.

# Personal health is more cost effective than illness

One study found that the cost of healthy eating is about $1.50 per day per person extra. We don't feel this is a valid excuse or argument to be made against ketogenic eating. There is a range of options in food costs that obviously can affect this daily cost. We believe the savings over time due to better health results will more than make up for this cost difference and is well worth the investment. This is simply another issue of mindset. We must retrain our thinking from "healthy is expensive" to "healthy is worth it."

One of many articles of interest to us takes a look at the 30,000-foot view of the costs of unhealthy eating and the price of the results on society. The question the article asks is this: "What drives poor health in America?"

The answer is simple: "Food is the **number one cause** of poor health in America."

Dietary habits, choices, and the systems that provide them are the leading driver of death and disability in America, causing an estimated 700,000 deaths each year. Heart disease, stroke, obesity, type 2 diabetes, cancers, immune function and brain health are all influenced and affected by what we eat. Recent research estimates that poor diet causes nearly half of all U.S. deaths due to heart disease, stroke and diabetes. Each day there are 1,000 deaths in the USA from these causes.

To put this into perspective you can easily understand, almost twice as many Americans are estimated to die each year as a result of poor dietary choices (58,000 deaths/year) than from car accidents (35,000/year).

Poor eating also contributes to disparities in the USA. People with lower incomes or otherwise disadvantaged often make the worst eating choices, causing a vicious cycle of poor health, lost productivity, increased health costs, and continued poverty.

Anything we can do to change this for one human being is worthy of our best efforts.

## The costs of poor dietary choices

Here is an undeniable, indisputable fact we feel bears repeating: **type 1 diabetics**, or those who have a pancreas that just does not produce insulin, account for a mere **5%** of those who use insulin.

The bad news is that **95%** of people using insulin are **type 2 diabetics.** The good news is that the vast majority of these human beings, millions of people, increasing in numbers by the millions each year, spending billions of dollars on insulin, are doing so by choice. Yes, we will keep repeating it. It is the truth.

If these people would simply make the choice to stop ingesting sugar, we believe as we have witnessed again and again as well as having experienced this on a deeply personal level, this huge and growing segment of the population would be able to greatly reduce or eliminate the medications they currently require to control their blood sugar.

This would be billions of dollars that could be put to a much more productive use. Please do not make the argument to us that eating healthy is expensive. We have witnessed the irrefutable truth. Once again this will be a mindset shift for most people. The amount of money we spend on healthcare each year is difficult to comprehend. The staggering number is between three and four trillion dollars per year. This represents 20% of all spending in the entire U.S. economy. This number represents about **$1,000 per month** for every man, woman, and child in America, exceeding most people's budget for food, gas, housing, and other common necessities.

The costs associated with poor dietary choices make up huge portions of this spending. Heart disease accounts for about

$200 billion in healthcare spending and another $125 billion in lost productivity and other indirect costs. The root cause of this spending is **sugar.**

Healthcare costs are crippling American businesses large and small. Ever increasing healthcare costs are major obstacles to growth and success. An amazing quote by business and investing legend Warren Buffett explains the situation perfectly. He described rising medical costs as the "tapeworm of American economic competitiveness." Our food system is feeding the tapeworm.

Remarkably, healthy eating and nutrition is practically ignored by our healthcare system. Healthcare has become politicized with the passing of Obamacare. Once again, the political system, no matter who you vote for, seems to focus on control and ignores the root cause of our current health issues in America. The reality is the vast majority of doctors get very little training in nutrition and even less on healthy eating during their education.

While this is true, we cannot miss the opportunity to express our gratitude to Dr. Jason Fung who we mentioned earlier, Dr. Eric Berg, and Dr. Ken D. Berry. These doctors, who in our humble opinion became humbly honest with themselves and became their own best educational advocates, realized formal education did not teach the whole truth about diet and nutrition or the overall health effects on human beings. We feel these are some of the pioneers who have gone against the grain and the system to truly help educate the public with truth. A sincere thank you for helping us save ourselves.

While we continue to see more in the medical field become enlightened to the nutritional reality of the education system, we must point out that most doctors seem to get out of medical school and into practice with a full understanding of how to prescribe the drugs that treat the symptoms of poor dietary choices and full knowledge of how that affects their compensation.

Another amazing statistic is that total federal spending across all agencies amounts to $1.5 billion per year. Industry spending on research for drugs, biotech, and medical devices totals $60 billion per year. This is *60 times* the spending by companies cashing in and profiting off the symptoms of poor dietary choices with *zero* attention being paid to the root cause of the issue and seemingly *zero* concern about the human toll this causes. The big wheel just keeps on turning. Kudos to those doctors and others in the medical field who are pushing forward with self-education rather than accepting the status quo.

We completely understand that the changes that need to be made would be difficult and require bipartisan support, during a time in American history in which the government has never appeared more divided. This does not cause the average ordinary person to hold out much hope that partisan bickering over irrelevant issues will make way for compromise that benefits the voters of America.

We believe the only way to force the issue is to continue sharing the ketogenic lifestyle, teaching what we have learned and getting results. Many doctors are starting to see the undeniable truth of hard facts with their patients. The results being demonstrated in real time speak louder than anything. One patient at a time, as irrefutable evidence in obesity, blood pressure, heart disease, and reversal of the symptoms of type 2 diabetes are being documented, and as the prescriptions these patients have been using to treat the symptoms of poor dietary choices are reduced or eliminated, we will reach a tipping point. We deeply believe this is happening.

The only way to destroy the powerful wheel that is keeping the masses trapped in the current system of sick care is to turn the wheel inside out and make the old system irrelevant. This is a huge task that we will continue to work on, one person at a time.

## Spending on healthcare now is a better investment than funding sick care in the future

The cost of healthier foods is relative. It is more of a short-term mindset change than anything. Buying healthy foods may cost a little more in the short term, but we have witnessed people that didn't think they could afford the cost change their mindset. They become unwilling to pay the price of sick care when they take an honest look.

By introducing intermittent fasting or time-based eating, many involved in the ketogenic lifestyle cut out a meal per day. The money saved by not eating this meal can be used to offset other costs or to add a supplement for testing. If your argument is that you eat off the dollar menu for breakfast, we will continue to repeat what we always say: the dollar menu mentality is what got many of us into the unhealthy condition of desperately needing the ketogenic lifestyle. We believe you are worth more than that.

Some things are changing at higher levels that are great for better health and wellness, and the perceived higher cost of eating healthier foods is changing. If we continue to add things, one at a time, to the system that offsets healthy choice costs or improves the average person's ability to get better nutritional information, we consider that small victories. This helps the mindset.

As we move into the era of electronic health records, adding the subject of nutrition to the system would be helpful. Insurance programs offering incentives for healthier eating would be a huge benefit. In fact, some life insurance companies are beginning to see the value and return on investment by rewarding clients for using health tracking devices or offering lower premiums and healthy food benefits which offset healthy nutrition costs up to $600 per year. These companies have determined through studies that every $1 spent on these type of wellness programs can return around $3 in lowered medical costs and absenteeism. If they would just recommend the minimization of sugar intake, they would save more than that.

We also suggest that instead of making healthy eating choices into an expense, to view the cost as an investment. Take an honest inventory of personal monthly spending and look for anything that can be replaced by more important choices of health and wellness. Commit to do a 30-, 60- or 90-day test and track your progress and results just as you would track your macros and food intake. You may find, like many of us have discovered, that the results and benefits received from the ketogenic lifestyle far outweigh the short-term thinking of cost.

We in no way want to minimize or ignore the fact that we have different spectrums of the economic ladder all over the world. We have been at the bottom of this ladder, and we have fought and clawed our way up that ladder at different periods of our lives. Our thinking was different at the bottom of the economic ladder than it is now, but some things only changed because we decided to change.

# CHAPTER 8

# Be Your Own Advocate/ Do Your Own Research

The vast majority of the food supply is controlled by 10 companies. This is not our opinion. This is a fact easily researched. Each of these companies owns and controls multiple brands. Each of those brands represents a multitude of products. The revenue from these companies in 2015 ranged from $13.5 billion on the low end to $90 billion at the high end. Altogether, these 10 companies accounted for approximately $837 billion of revenue.

We don't think it would be outside of the realm of possibility that these companies know a thing or two about marketing. Add to these 10 companies those who represent fast food and we add another $463 billion of revenue.

They may know a thing or two about marketing as well. We will discuss some of the tactics they use that cause you to think about and crave their "food" even when you are not even hungry. It almost seems like black magic or sorcery of some sort, but considering the never-ending barrage of advertising we are subjected to every waking hour on every form of media, the message is implanted in our psyche.

These companies are well aware of our pain points. We seem to always be in a rush, under stress for many reasons, and the choice with the least possible friction is most often the nearest drive-through window. There are over 200,000 fast food restaurants in the U.S. and this amounts to having a readily available pit stop for food in just about any small town and at least within driving distance of most people. So convenient and so fast!

Fast food companies take advantage of the average person's desire for convenience. Over the past few decades we have been psychologically trained to value convenience over health. These fast foods are designed to trigger the pleasure centers of the brain despite the fact they are devoid of healthy nutrition.

The **average** fast food meal is approximately **1,000 calories**. This is before super-sizing or value-sizing. Please keep in mind that the average soda serving has increased from seven to 32 ounces over the last four decades, and the size of French fry servings has nearly tripled from 2.4 ounces to 5.4 ounces. This is before super-sizing that order. It is easy to see how the average person consuming fast food is taking in entirely too many calories per day. If we are so busy that we must choose a drive-through, we are probably too busy to worry about counting calories.

It is no secret that fast food chains target their advertising at children. In a 2009 study by Yale University, it was estimated that $4.2 billion was spent by fast food chains on advertising. The study found that preschoolers saw an increase in ads for fast food ranging from about 9% to as high as 56%, and children aged 6 to 11 saw even higher numbers as compared with 2007 data. You, your children and your grandchildren are *targets*.

There is also the subject of *secret ingredients*, trade secrets that make each brand special. What about hidden ingredients and chemicals that never make it on to the menu or nutrition guide? Many of these companies have so much chemical garbage, preservatives and additives that most people cannot pronounce, much less understand what they are and what side effects might be caused from eating them. They don't want you to know.

Isn't that just amazing? That "all natural" order of fries that sounds so much healthier actually contains up to 19 different ingredients, most we cannot pronounce, that are anything but healthy.

The slippery slope gets even worse when we start looking at other "healthy" descriptions that companies use like "fat free," "low fat," "sugar free," and "no sugar added." The definitions get really complicated, and we believe that is done on purpose to murk up the waters as much as possible.

Compared to 30 years ago, an average cheeseburger can contain as much as 75% more calories. The average order of fries is almost 200% more calories. The average slice of pizza is 70% more calories. This is due to a combination of increased portion sizes and ingredient choices. The average milkshake exceeds the daily recommended allowance of sugar by two to three times. Add one to your already super-sized meal and your calories can exceed what you should consume in a day.

If you choose to become self-educated on the subject of marketing and advertising tricks used by the big food companies and the fast food companies, it is upsetting. Not only is it upsetting to see how this kind of marketing affects us personally and the choices we make, but when we see the impact it is having on our children and grandchildren we feel sickened. To deeply understand the level of control these companies are exerting by focusing on marketing directly to children should be seriously alarming.

Unfortunately, it appears the responsibility for protecting our kids from this system of control is falling on the shoulders of the parents and grandparents of these kids, the very people who have been subjected to these practices in marketing and advertising for decades.

Ian and Betsy attempted a discussion with their 12-year-old granddaughter. The subject of making healthier choices or discussing the amount of sugar and processed ingredients went over like a lead balloon. She was only concerned that she is hungry *now*, and she knows exactly what she wants and exactly where to get it. Exactly the way we have been marketed and trained. Mission accomplished, fast food industry.

Despite attempting to have a rational conversation about healthy food, this beautiful young girl, who loves dance and animals, simply does not want to hear about this issue. We worry about her future. We do the best we can at home to feed her healthy foods, but if left to her own choices, the psychological training and marketing she has experienced in her life causes her to act exactly the way a fast food company would want.

# CHAPTER 9

# Open Your Mind to Learn New Things

For Ian, becoming open minded to learn new things took a threat to his employment and livelihood. For Jim, it was losing most of his right foot to amputation due to symptoms of diabetes that got his attention. Both Ian and Jim were obese and unhealthy. We are suggesting that you have the power of choice and do not have to go to these extremes to make an amazing turnaround in your health and weight right now.

Our hope and goal of this book is that you become awakened right now. You can make an honest assessment of your current health. You can take a look back at the journey that brought you to this point. For most people, this personal inventory and examination of the honest facts should be all it takes to make a decision to take responsibility for their own health and wellness. It does not have to get to the point of a health crisis before this decision is made.

If you are in a health crisis or situation where you are feeling that there is no hope, we want to encourage you to just get started. We have witnessed so many dramatic and amazing transformations and turnarounds with people's health that we *expect* it.

The good news is this:

No matter how many decades it has taken you to get to the point that you are willing to read this book, the very act of opening your mind to some new and different information to simply get started in a new direction is a start.

Think of it this way: if it has taken three, four, or even five decades to get your weight or health to the point that you are willing to read this book, so what if it took a single year to get yourself to your goal weight?

This really puts into perspective the healing power of the ketogenic lifestyle. We have the power to literally reverse decades of sugar overconsumption in a relatively short period of time. We do not recommend setting a goal of losing more than one pound per week. This makes the math very simple. Set this in your mind from the beginning. Make up your mind that you are going to be here in a year. You are worthy of your very best effort.

One of the realities that we came to realize is a simple universal truth: you don't know what you don't know. The only way to change this is to become open minded to some new and better information. There is now an overwhelming amount of information to choose from. We just don't know what we don't know. We would like to share some perspective of how things have changed over the past 25 years.

Ian was given a book for his birthday around the year of 1995 by his sister Julie. The book was *Dr. Atkins New Diet Revolution*. This would be what we call a clue when your family member gives you a book because she is concerned about your weight! The point is that until that moment I had never even heard of the Atkins diet (a low-carb/higher protein diet than ketogenic). The book was originally published in 1972, and I had never heard of it.

Here are some things that have totally changed since then:

In 1995, Windows 95 was just released. The internet had just been born. Smartphones didn't exist. It took 10 minutes for a picture off the internet to upload on your computer screen. To connect to the internet, we used things called dial-up modems. Cable modems did not exist, and barely anyone but college students or the military even knew how to navigate the internet.

Most people got their media from the newspapers, magazines and the local and national nightly news. If those sources didn't cover something or think it was important, we didn't hear about it.

Access to this type of information that is instant today was not available back in 1995. In fact, today we are bombarded to the point of continuous overwhelm at all times. In these modern times of 24-hour news cycle, continuous political broadcasting, and the age of smartphones with continuous access to the internet, we now face the opposite problem.

There is more information available to the average human through the computational power of a smartphone connected to the internet now than at any time in human history. It seems as if every possible subject can be taken from one extreme to the other, and there is information available covering every possible angle.

"Confusing," "overwhelming" and "discouraging" are all words we have heard from our members who just want to know where to start. They just want to know the basics so they can begin to take one step forward at a time in the right direction. This can seem impossible when many different gurus on a topic disagree and seem to talk over each other to get attention and be heard. We understand that and acknowledge that this is the current reality new people face when getting started with the ketogenic lifestyle.

Ian was given a book. That was the sum total of all information about low-carb dieting that he had ever heard of in his life. The book did not prepare him for electrolyte imbalance or dealing with the symptoms of the keto flu, and blood ketone meters did not even exist. Ian was introduced to urine strips that would display a color change in the presence of ketones being expelled in the urine. There was no conflicting information or differences of opinion. There was simply a single book to go by.

What is interesting to reflect on is that as this "fad diet" gained some popularity and news coverage back in those days, most people that Ian knew that tried the Atkins diet never even read the book. The *one* book that was available.

Having now worked with tens of thousands of people, Ian sees a striking similarity as new people start the ketogenic lifestyle today. Even with the staggering amount of information, conflicting opinions of gurus and experts, and the internet at our fingertips, many people just blindly jump into what they think is the ketogenic lifestyle based off what they have heard.

That is exactly what many people did back then. They simply cut out carbs the best they knew how and started eating meat, eggs, cheese, and salad. There was no information about electrolyte imbalance, keto flu, or any suggestions of how to minimize these side effects of eating low carb. These negative consequences were just the price to be paid to enter the low-carb lifestyle and also the single issue to cause most people to fail, in our opinion.

What is interesting is that today, with more information available in the smartphone everyone carries around connected to the internet, we see the same thing occurring with many people starting the ketogenic lifestyle. We believe this is caused by the overabundance of information, much of it conflicting or confusing, that causes people to attempt to just go it alone.

Some people tend to just get started without any or very little guidance, and they are dealing with the same issues of electrolyte imbalance and keto flu that caused so many to fail and quit in the past. Our goal is to change that by offering some simple steps to get started the right way by educating on some simple things to do or supplements to take to minimize or eliminate the keto flu and provide the average person with a guide to better success.

We understand this amazing abundance of information and opinions is available. Some of it will still be available when you have successfully started the ketogenic lifestyle, and the new person can make a personal choice of who they trust to get the best information from.

We both do a lot of research. As our minds and eyes have been opened to the history of nutrition, the pharmaceutical industry, the education system, medical establishment, and the government's role in all of it, it can be difficult not to get upset, and we have been as careful as we can that this book not just turn into a rant or just another conspiracy theory.

We have spent a great many hours of our lives digging into books, articles, and other information using the power of the internet. We are always aware to consider the angles that all of the different writers of information are coming from. What might be the motivation?

One thing becomes very clear with the amount of time we have spent, and the amount of energy put into researching and reading for our own personal understanding and education: there are many agendas out there in the world. We simply suggest that you stay aware of this and keep your eyes open to this.

"Follow the money" is a phrase we have all heard. When we uncover the history of business manipulating the educational system, government policy and the medical community, it can cause us to wonder if we can believe anyone at all. Money has shown the power to influence studies to produce the desired outcome instead of the truth. This does not help people become healthier.

The information is out there. We can learn from history. It is our hope and goal that we can actually make a positive change in the health of people that seek it. This will require the truth. It will require results. It will happen one person at a time.

The final part of this chapter will include certain associations that exist in America, supposedly for the purpose of promoting health and wellness. They speak with authority and put their stamp of approval on products. Many of these associations exist, including those representing heart disease and diabetes as a couple of examples. There are many good people that volunteer for organizations like this, and we have no issue with any of these good people. We do have a problem with the system.

These "associations" are charities. Follow the money. Understand where the money comes from and it answers so many questions. When esteemed associations have toed the company line that fat is unhealthy and that we should eat more carbohydrates, and the end results of this policy is an explosion of heart disease, obesity and diabetes, we must follow the money. It comes from big food companies, big drug companies and lobby groups for competing interests of the ketogenic way of eating.

When an association like this takes an official stance that coconut oil is unhealthy despite an overwhelming amount of evidence that any reasonable person can understand, we start to realize associations like this are just another spoke in the wheel of the giant sugar machine. The fact that associations put their heart healthy stamp of approval on breakfast cereals full of sugar makes any recommendation they make irrelevant. How can they even be taken seriously? Instead, they reveal themselves to be just another manipulation of the big money system that is ultimately not promoting better long-term health for the public.

Here is another couple of examples of a major nationwide association dealing with blood sugar and issues involving following the money:

"In May of 2006, The Philadelphia Inquirer reported that (this association) had 'privately enlisted an Eli Lilly & Company executive to chart its growth strategy and write its slogan. Lilly executive ----- Jr. told the Inquirer that he helped the organization market itself and came up with its slogan, 'Cure. Care. Commitment.' He estimated his work would have cost 'hundreds of thousands' from a contractor." (Sourcewatch.org)

"Also, the Inquirer reported that the 'association' did not include in its 2000-2001 annual report that Hall had been seconded into the organization. ----, it reported, moved into its Alexandria, Va., headquarters and coached it on growth strategies, all paid by Lilly."

The vice president for development, for the 'association' said, "We always walk a fine line on showing favoritism to one company over another. I would imagine other corporate donors would look askance at it." She also added if it were offered again, "we'd ask for money." Just as a friendly reminder of who Eli Lilly & Co. is – a pharmaceutical company that happens to manufacture and sell Humalog insulin, among many other products.

Finally, we offer this case in point:

"If you are wondering why Americans are losing the wars on cancer, heart disease and diabetes you might look at the funding sources of the major public health groups," Russell Mokiber and Robert Weissman wrote in May of 2005. "Big corporations dump big money into these groups. And pretty soon, the groups start taking the line of the big corporations."

Another case in point:

"The 'association' (dealing with blood sugar) earlier in the month, had cut a deal with candy and soda pop maker ------ who kicked in a *couple million dollars* to the 'association' and in return gets to use the 'association' label on its diet drinks. Plus, the positive publicity generated by the deal. You would have to have your head buried deeply in the sand to deny that sugar filled soda is fueling childhood obesity, and in turn fueling type 2 diabetes." (Sourcewatch.org)

Once again, there are so many examples of this that we could write another book. We only want you to understand the system we are dealing with when it comes to these trusted associations who claim to be looking out for the public. The truth is they are looking out for their organization and the partners that dump the millions in funding.

It is not a giant leap of understanding that they have a vested interest in maintaining the growth and profits of those corporate partners. It seems "Joe Public" doesn't really have anyone looking out for his personal health. Our suggestion is he better take the responsibility to be his own advocate.

One final thought we want to share is to urge you to make use of the internet and the search engine of your choice. Search for answers to questions that pop up. Practice this until you get good at locating good sources of information. Learning to search for the answer of "Can I eat... on keto?" is literally a few clicks and seconds instead of asking someone else. Nutrition labels and ingredients are readily available for most foods.

## A note on intermittent fasting

We both practice intermittent fasting. We came across the topic while on our own individual keto journeys, put it into practice, and decided that it was something that fit perfectly into the new lifestyle we each were building. We also discovered that like the ketogenic lifestyle and many other topics, there are different opinions and extremist views from one end of the spectrum to the other.

For the purposes of this book, we will discuss intermittent fasting as time-based eating, or taking in personal macro and calorie requirements during a window of time each day. Most people are simply stopping food intake by 8pm and then not eating again until noon the next day. We have found the combination of ketogenic lifestyle with intermittent fasting to be a powerful complementary combination that provides great health benefits and synergies.

Intermittent fasting changes cellular function as well as the function of genes and hormones. Some of these changes can include lower insulin levels. This is really helpful in burning fat. Human growth hormone may increase as much as five times facilitating muscle growth and fat burn. The body can induce cellular repair processes and remove waste material from cells.

There are beneficial changes in several genes and molecules related to longevity and protection against disease.

Intermittent fasting aids in weight loss by eating fewer meals and enhancing hormone function to facilitate weight loss. Lower insulin levels, increased human growth hormone, and increased amounts of norepinephrine (noradrenaline) all increase breakdown of body fat to use for energy.

For this reason, short-term fasting actually increases the metabolic rate 3.6-14% helping to burn more calories. According to scientific literature, intermittent fasting can cause weight loss of 3-8% over 3-24 weeks.

Intermittent fasting can reduce insulin resistance and lower type 2 diabetes risk. Intermittent fasting can reduce oxidative stress and inflammation in the body. Intermittent fasting has been shown to improve multiple risk factors for heart disease. Autophagy or cellular repair and waste removal may provide protection against such disease as cancer and Alzheimer's disease.

Intermittent fasting is good for the brain and improves various metabolic features known to aid brain health. These neuro-protective properties combined with increases in lifespan are benefits that make combining intermittent fasting with the ketogenic lifestyle extremely powerful.

This basic introduction to intermittent fasting should be enough information to make you understand that this powerful combination is worth getting educated about and put into practice for a few months. This should be enough time to decide if intermittent fasting is right for you. We strongly suggest you do some research and put this practice to the test for a long enough time period to see actual results.

In our First Steps 2 Keto 30-Day Challenge we actually work with people each month of the challenge to implement intermittent fasting. We answer questions that come up and work individually with each person to fit this into the ketogenic lifestyle. The results have been fantastic, and we love to see members working with their doctors as they reduce, minimize and eliminate medications that are no longer needed.

# CHAPTER 10

# Ketogenic Lifestyle at Home and on the Road

The ketogenic lifestyle is really a major shift in mindset. When we open our minds to new and better information, and take an honest look at the information that has been taught to us, any normal person should have no issue with understanding the misinformation we have been exposed to since childhood is wrong, and we have to choose to reprogram what we know to be the truth.

If our body's blood sugar control system is not functioning properly, we must come to the realization that we cannot keep ingesting what our system will not control. We regularly see new people getting started into the ketogenic lifestyle who ask, "When do I get a cheat meal?" What they are really asking is, "When do I get to ingest sugar again?"

We have a couple of points to make. You are not a dog or some kind of circus animal that gets rewarded with treats for doing good. The behavior is simply self-sabotage. The faster you can remove this old thinking pattern and develop a better mindset, the less likely you will have to suffer the negative consequences of self-sabotaging your progress with negative behavior that serves zero positive purpose. If you are going to set a goal, consider shopping for new clothes because the big clothes you used to wear no longer fit you. We never recommend rewarding yourself with food.

The only response to any choice or option about what we put in our body should be: Is this choice going to bring me closer to my goal in a positive way, or take me farther away? The choice will never be about deserving to eat sugar. We do recommend learning to make some amazing keto friendly desserts, bread, or pasta that proves to yourself that you can still eat amazing foods that taste good. All that you are really giving up is poisoning yourself with sugar.

The choice we all have will be about taking responsibility for self-care, and not allowing short-term cravings or old negative thinking to derail our progress. The only way to create new habits is to practice the new behavior. Anything in life that we want to improve will require practice. The more we practice, the better we will get at making better healthier choices. There will be times when we are alone and nobody would know but us. These are the times that count. The times when nobody would even know. This is when we must practice the positive habit of integrity. We only have integrity when we are the same person who makes the right choices even when nobody else is looking.

There will be times when we are on the road, traveling, running late, or on vacation. We may decide to finally go on that cruise. You know the one: the cruise with all you can eat everything, anytime you want it. We all will be faced with these situations. It is always better to have thought things through ahead of time.

*Failing to plan is planning to fail.*

The unexpected can happen at any time during times of travel and out on the road. It is always better to have planned ahead than it is to have to react when hungry and stressed. Simple choices to plan ahead to prepare for anything that happens that is unexpected is the best plan. Our health is our responsibility, not someone else's. We have lived that life thinking it was someone else that was in charge of it, and that didn't work out well.

Having your own keto approved snacks while traveling makes a huge difference if plans get upset. Cancelled flights, hotel problems, or transportation problems can and do pop up at inconvenient times. It is worth repeating as it is so important to understand. Failing to plan is planning to fail. We choose to be ready if the situation changes.

Going to parties and gatherings is another time to plan ahead. Bring your own keto approved snacks and just put them on the same plates everyone else is using. Don't make a big deal out of it, and people most probably won't even know. We don't have to make a big deal about it or draw attention to ourselves. We are simply taking care of ourselves. It is not the host's responsibility to understand our personal health issues.

Going out to restaurants can be a total unknown. As you practice the ketogenic lifestyle and start testing blood ketone levels with a meter, it is good to practice at local restaurants to question the waiter. Let them know you are eating ketogenic. So many more people are eating this way that many restaurants are responding by providing keto or at least low-carb options. Not knowing the ingredients used can make this a minefield. We would recommend testing blood ketone levels before and 30 minutes to an hour after eating at a restaurant. This is the only way to know if they slipped something into a recipe or are using a salad dressing high in carbs. Be your own advocate and never assume. Assuming is just not an effective strategy.

Family gatherings can be another interesting event to plan for. Family members can be some of the most difficult people to deal with. They will say things other people won't because they are family. I will refer you back to the crabs in a bucket analogy. As you are climbing out of the bucket of poor health and bad food choices, there will be others in your life that don't have the same level of information or desire to change.

They don't mind you getting better, just not better than them. Like crabs in a bucket, they will pull you back down to their level. You must be mentally prepared for this to come from some of the most unexpected people. They will be more than willing to share their totally uneducated and misinformed opinions with you. Arguing with them or attempting to change their mind is usually an exhausting waste of time and energy. They don't know what they don't know.

Be prepared, don't argue, and the truth is that the ketogenic lifestyle is strong enough that it doesn't need any of us to stand up for it. Thank them for their input and concern and go about your business. Let your ongoing success be the noise. Your results will speak louder than any facts you can argue. Nothing gets results like results.

Always be ready to tell yourself, "Isn't that interesting?" when you witness or experience a family member or friend act this way. Your results will be what changes people's minds to want to know what you are doing. It is so much easier to share your experience coming from that place of proven results.

It is also a good idea to set expectations in advance when needed. We cannot cover every possible scenario for this, but it is always in your best interest to plan ahead for any event instead of having to react to a bad situation.

Do not allow anyone to guilt or shame you into eating things you know will not contribute to your progress. You are worthy of better treatment than to take that behavior from anyone. Anyone who fails to give you the respect you deserve to take control of your personal health and wellness has done you a great favor. They have let you know that they are someone you don't need to be around.

This is a lifestyle, not a diet, and the lifestyle requires a shift in mindset. In our opinion, the ketogenic lifestyle is 95% mindset and

5% eating ketogenic food. As we continue to expand our personal education and practice the positive behaviors of the ketogenic lifestyle, it will get easier. The choices become more automatic with practice. We start to become unconsciously competent in making the right choices where before, when just getting started, we were unconsciously incompetent. We just did not know what we did not know. It takes practice.

We hope this information provided is enough to build your belief that you can make this change for your life and health if you simply get started. There is no possible way to cover every scenario and provide the answer to every single possible question in this book. What we discovered for ourselves is that if you become open to better information, you have the absolute ability to find the solution that works best for you. This is what being your own best advocate is all about. The willingness to find the best solution for you is the key to transitioning successfully into the ketogenic lifestyle.

# CHAPTER 11

# Final Thoughts and Information: Where this Journey is Taking Us!

A word of caution. Nobody likes a know-it-all. Worse than a know-it-all is the person we refer to as the "keto-extremist." This is the know-it-all who takes it to the next level.

This is the person who starts spewing keto information on people who have not requested it, nor even care to hear about it. Think about how you feel about some random person giving unsolicited advice on any topic. It is no different than the keto-extremist who tells everyone what they should and shouldn't eat, as well as what kind of potential damage they are doing to themselves and/or their children.

We remember feeling alone when we got our start into this lifestyle, we were seeking out information, and wanting to belong to a group of people practicing the same lifestyle for the same reasons. We felt that there is power in a group. As we checked options on social media, what we ran into over and over were these keto-extremists.

We found people giving unsolicited advice, telling people what they should be doing and even degrading new people for asking the questions that new people ask. We witnessed certain keto-extremists tell people that certain things were and were not keto, things like diet soda that has zero carbs, because it has artificial sweeteners in it. We found people taking extremist views on all manner of subjects, and frankly, some of this defied explanation.

So, we just decided to start our own group. We decided that there would be certain behaviors that we just would not tolerate. We decided that new people would be our focus. We wanted to help them get started in the right way. We decided we would not tolerate anyone being talked down to or belittled. We wanted people to feel comfortable and get their questions answered.

We decided to do our best to anchor our belief system firmly in the middle of the extremist views that range from one spectrum to the other. From "lazy keto" that we believe produces the laziest results, to the hard-core keto-extremist who views anything with a carb as poison (yes, we have seen and met them), we believe we are on middle ground.

We discovered that culture and community are really important in this lifestyle. While some people are loners and comfortable going it alone, so many more of us crave and thrive on community. So, we built it. We imagined it, we prayed about it, and we just went to work and built an amazing community. As the community has grown, we have run into every kind of limitation from personal growth limitations, technology limitations, and even time limitations. Despite all this, the group continued to grow.

We must acknowledge that there are now many amazing groups that have grown over time that are bringing amazing value to the keto community. Some of the doctors mentioned previously have Facebook groups as well as amazing video content. We have some amazing friends in the keto space who have helped us learn about groups, social media, and automation technology that is helping us share what we have learned with more people, as well as learn to use social media in a better more responsible way. Thank you to all who have helped make us better.

We do our best to provide information to the newest person to help them get started, despite the limitations of social media. We simply keep focused on finding better ways to get the message to more people. As the community has grown, so has engagement, and so much so that it is now very difficult to make sure that all the members of the community receive all the information. In the age of email showing lower and lower open rates, this also proved a challenge as we could not rely on emails to get the information to everyone.

This has led us to chatbot technology, or as we now call it Keto-bot technology. We now have the ability to deliver specific content, training and encouragement to each person who decides to join our group. We have the ability to provide the newest person with the proper steps to get started correctly and to share with them the mistakes we have seen new people make so they don't have to repeat them. We can deliver meal plans, content for training, ask questions, and allow for input from the member, and this increases engagement in a way that email never did.

We were doing a live video sharing some experience we had learned one day and Jim said, "We should do a 30-Day Challenge and teach anyone who wants to learn the things that we have put into practice that has gotten us our health back." Jim blurted it out, just like that.

When the video was over, we connected on Zoom, a video conferencing app, and we went to work mapping out what a 30-Day Challenge would look like.

What Jim didn't know is that a month before, while in Knoxville, Tennessee, Ian had been brainstorming about how to better help the new person get started in the ketogenic lifestyle. It really came down to the question, "What are the first steps to keto?" He had been thinking more and more about taking those first steps. Ian decided to check for the domain name FirstSteps2Keto.com and found that it was available and purchased it without really having a plan for what to do with it.

A month later, we started mind mapping what a 30-Day Challenge would look like, consist of, and what we would want to share with the newest person getting started. That is how the idea of First Steps 2 Keto came to be, from a simple thought, to an idea, to a collaboration.

It was during these conversations that the idea of writing a book came up. It was something that we had both separately thought about wanting to do. We looked at each other and just decided the time was now. We made a decision.

We hired a coach and just got started. We took advice and coaching from someone with more experience than we had. We followed instructions and trusted in the experience of our coach. This connection is one of the most important decisions we have made as the book you are holding in your hand is the result of a couple of regular guys who had some extraordinary experiences, and made some major lifestyle changes. The point of sharing this is that we are following the same process of change.

We stopped thinking about it, we made a decision to get started, and we learned from others with more experience. **We got started**.

We wanted to share this bit of our history with you for a couple of different reasons. We have been where you are. We failed at multiple attempts at so many different types of diets that it pains us to look back on it. We both had no real expectation to succeed with the ketogenic lifestyle. We had been conditioned to fail at one more thing. It was normal.

The difference this time for both of us is that we just decided we were ready as the new information came into our lives and consciousness. There really is not a better way to describe what happened or what was different. At some point, we just made the decision that we were ready, and this time was different.

For the first part of our individual journeys, we were really selfish in the sense that we focused on ourselves. We focused on cleaning up our own mess and putting into practice those new ideas and concepts that we needed to be successful, for ourselves.

We didn't turn into know-it-alls and put the focus on telling everyone else what they needed to do or change. The information we relied upon was the problem and we spent our time getting better information to improve ourselves. We became students of the process and really put the things that worked for us into practice. We let go of the things that did not work for us with no hard feelings. It was just a part of the process, and as we have previously mentioned, there was so much information, so many competing voices talking over each other to be heard, so many differences of opinion that we really didn't know who to listen to or where the best information was available. We did the trial and error method and fortunately were able to continue to make progress.

Over time, other people who know us started seeing the results of what we were doing. Some of those people made comments of congratulations, but some people wanted information. Some of them wanted coaching. They wanted someone to show them the way.

Both Ian and Jim had a struggle with wondering if we should be the ones to show these people the way. We had each individually been through the trial and error process, and we agreed that there had to be a better way that would provide more people with success.

The bottom line is that we had to take responsibility for helping ourselves heal and improve and get better educated before we could help others. Now that we made the decision to work together for the purpose of getting the new person started into the ketogenic lifestyle, we are finding out that reaching out to support other people in improving their personal health and wellness has been one of the very best things we have ever done to help ourselves.

Getting personal health and wellness back has been a huge benefit, but the feeling of satisfaction that we get as we witness more and more people that we work with getting healthy, reducing or eliminating medications, working through life traumas that have always been used as excuses to *not* take care of themselves, has been an amazing blessing.

To get to witness the ripple effect as many of these people begin leading by example and leading their own family and friends to better health and wellness has been some of the most gratifying experiences of our lives.

Jim didn't realize that people were silently watching his progress, including those that had made negative comments in the beginning. We like to say that nothing gets results like results, and Jim was getting stronger and healthier by the day. This is proof that by taking responsibility for your own personal health and wellness, you can become a powerful testimony to those who are watching your progress.

Jim's father is 74 years old and has had open heart surgery and has been an insulin dependent diabetic for over 20 years, as well as using Metformin and several other medications. Jim's mom was watching his progress slowly and began to wonder if this ketogenic lifestyle might help her and her husband. Although Jim's dad was resistant at first, Jim's mom persisted in slowly bringing them into the ketogenic way of eating. Mom started doing her own research and got better educated.

Jim's father began to experience the same health turnaround that his son did. As the sugar was cut back, his body began the healing process. Even after the heart surgery and all the medications he was on, his body started healing and the medications started being reduced and eliminated. He has continued to improve until he is now off all blood sugar medications.

Twenty years of dependence on insulin stopped, simply by removing sugar. Jim's dad, whom he was extremely concerned about after the heart surgery, is now wanting to get back in the gym. He was told that type 2 diabetes was a progressive and lifelong disease. We think the medical profession should be required to add an asterisk * Only if you choose to keep eating sugar.

Ian wanted to include this story. He didn't get a second chance with his dad, and to see Jim have the opportunity for more quality time with his dad is deeply gratifying. We would both desire for this to happen for many more people.

Once again, we point out that treating the symptoms of dietary choice with medication is not actually dealing with the root cause of the problem. The root cause is SUGAR. We are eternally grateful for witnessing these results with personal family members.

Ian, who lost his father at a very young age, is especially thankful to get to witness results like this. Anyone who gets to spend a little more time with those they love makes anything we have gone through absolutely worth it.

We have now worked together as a team, just a couple of regular guys who followed the Standard American Diet. We ate the food pyramid hook, line and sinker and ended up obese, with high blood pressure, heart issues, and diagnosed type 2 diabetic. Exactly the same results as about 95% of other humans eating the western diet.

We have taken this experience, become our own health and wellness advocates, done our research and are now living examples of what is possible. As people began to see the results in us, we started sharing what we have learned with others.

Something we have started offering is a FREE 7-Day Bootcamp. We offer this for people to get a good taste of what we are doing and teaching in our 30-Day Challenge.

Get started at bootcamp2.firststeps2keto.com

We also decided we wanted to do whatever we can to make a bigger impact. We have taken what we have learned, discussed it, mapped it out, and condensed it into some simple getting started steps. We created a 30-Day Challenge to teach the basics of ketogenic eating and intermittent fasting. We provide a meal plan, grocery lists and recipes. We also teach about figuring macros, tracking food intake, supplements, hormones, ketones, ketosis, and testing for ketones.

We do fun weekly giveaways, daily posts in our private challenge group, and weekly Coffee Talk Zoom calls where we meet up "face-to-face" on a teleconferencing app, share a cup of coffee or hot chocolate, and answer any questions from our members. We celebrate victories and encourage each other.

We are teaching and training our challenge members to be mentors to the next group of new people. We are developing a core group of raving fans who love the process and are paying it forward. If you have any interest in seeing for yourself if this is for you, please visit us at www.firststeps2keto.com for more information. We are focusing on supporting the newest person just getting started and teaching them the basics of the ketogenic lifestyle and intermittent fasting.

We call it the First Steps 2 Keto I/F 30-Day Challenge. You are invited.

# About the Authors

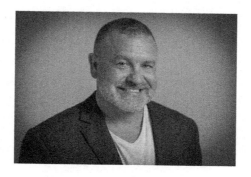

## Ian R. Prather

Ian Prather spent 25 years working 12-hour rotating shift work getting heavier every year. He reclaimed his health and opened a gym. He is co-founder of two popular Facebook groups on the ketogenic lifestyle. Social media has been the platform to impact many more people than working with clients one-on-one in a gym setting.

Ian has found a calling with a focus on helping the newest person get better educated on the role that overconsumption of sugar plays in our health and wellness. Having personally struggled through this process, being able to provide better information as well as avoiding common mistakes, is increasing positive results.

Now working from home full-time while supportive of his wife's career at NASA, Ian and his wife currently call the Houston, Texas area home and dream of making Arizona the home of their retirement. You can visit Ian R. Prather on Facebook.

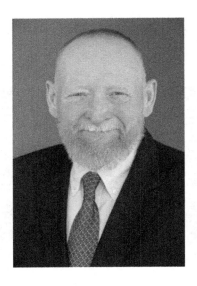

## Jim Withers

Jim Withers grew up an Air Force "brat," moving from base to base as a child. In 1976, his family settled in Galt, California where he graduated high school in 1983.

Jim joined the U.S. Navy in 1986 where he served for 13 years. He is a Gulf War combat Veteran, honorably discharged in 1998. After serving in the Navy, he became interested in sales and worked for many different corporations selling insurance, cars, and pest control. During this time, he did not pay attention to his diet and developed type 2 diabetes. In 2016, he lost the front of his right foot to amputation. By utilizing the ketogenic lifestyle, he is medication free and healthy.

Jim lives with his wife and childhood sweetheart Tammy Chappell Withers in Galt, California. They have three small dogs and numerous cats. Jim loves sharing his experiences and helping others learn the ketogenic lifestyle.

Made in the USA
Monee, IL
17 November 2019